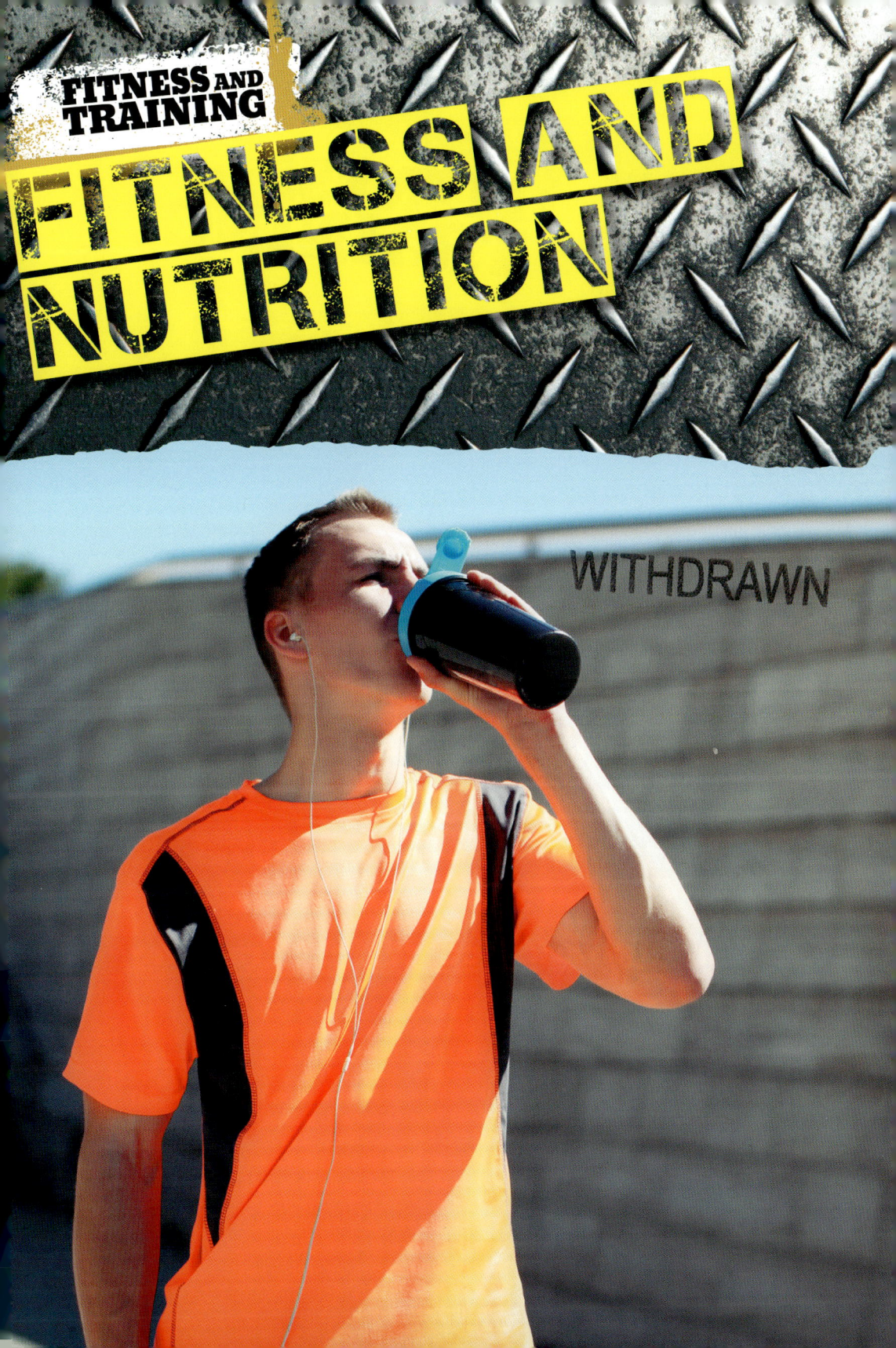

FITNESS AND TRAINING

Core Training
Endurance Training
Fitness and Nutrition
High-Energy Workouts
High-Intensity Interval Training (HIIT)
Low Impact Training
Mind and Body Fitness
Strength and Bodyweight Training

FITNESS AND TRAINING

FITNESS AND NUTRITION

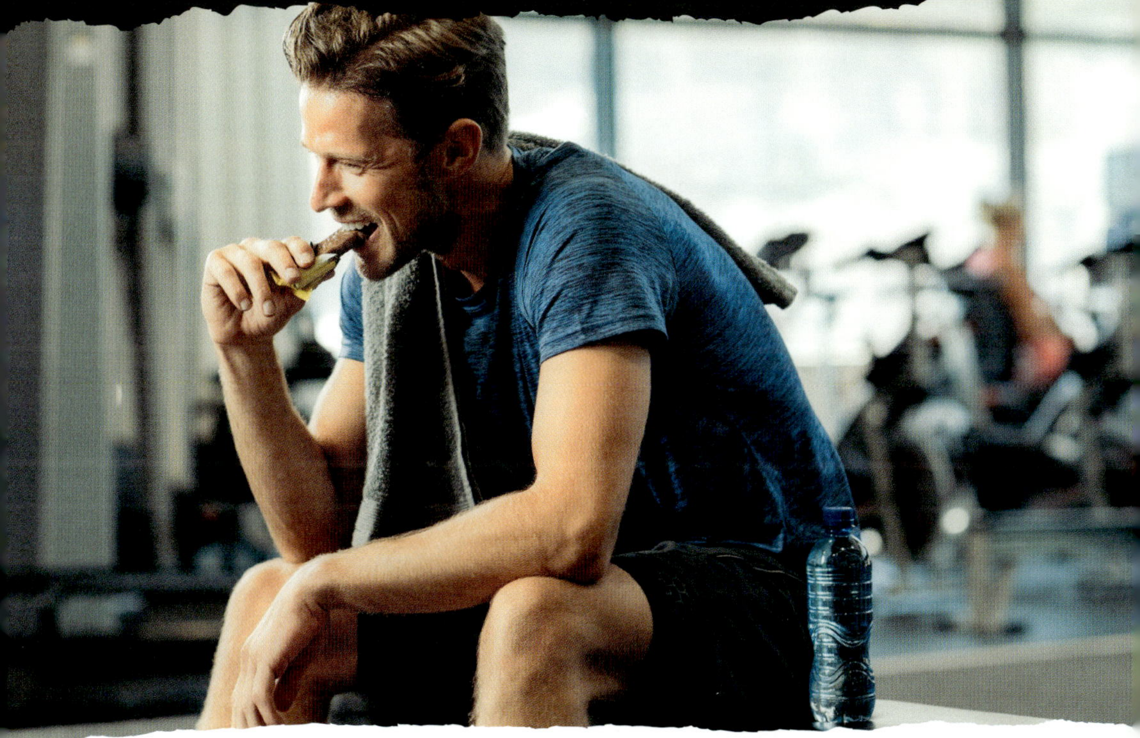

Kimber Rozier

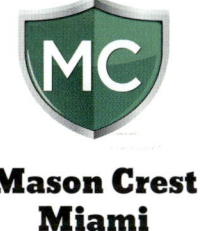

Mason Crest
Miami

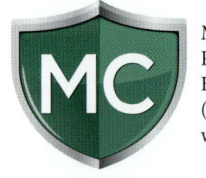

Mason Crest
PO Box 221876
Hollywood, FL 33022
(866) MCP-BOOK (toll-free)
www.masoncrest.com

Copyright © 2023 by Mason Crest, an imprint of National Highlights, Inc. All rights reserved. No part of this publication may be reproduced or transmitted in any form or by any means, electronic or mechanical, including photocopying, recording, taping, or any information storage and retrieval system, without permission from the publisher.

First printing
9 8 7 6 5 4 3 2 1
ISBN (hardback) 978-1-4222-4597-2
ISBN (series) 978-1-4222-4594-1
ISBN (ebook) 978-1-4222-7213-8

Library of Congress Cataloging-in-Publication Data

Names: Rozier, Kimber, author.
Title: Fitness and nutrition / Kimber Rozier.
Description: Hollywood, FL : Mason Crest, 2023 |
  Series: Fitness and training | Includes bibliographical references and index.
Identifiers: LCCN 2020009701 | ISBN 9781422245972 (hardback) |
  ISBN 9781422272138 (ebook)
Subjects: LCSH: Physical fitness–Juvenile literature. |
  Nutrition–Juvenile literature. | Health–Juvenile literature.
Classification: LCC RA781 .R699 2021 | DDC 613.7–dc23
LC record available at https://lccn.loc.gov/2020009701

Developed and Produced by National Highlights, Inc.
Editor: Andrew Luke
Production: Crafted Content, LLC

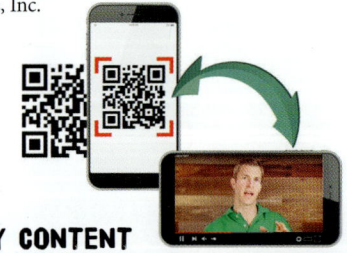

QR CODES AND LINKS TO THIRD-PARTY CONTENT

You may gain access to certain third-party content ("Third-Party Sites") by scanning and using the QR Codes that appear in this publication (the "QR Codes"). We do not operate or control in any respect any information, products, or services on such Third-Party Sites linked to by us via the QR Codes included in this publication, and we assume no responsibility for any materials you may access using the QR Codes. Your use of the QR Codes may be subject to terms, limitations, or restrictions set forth in the applicable terms of use or otherwise established by the owners of the Third-Party Sites. Our linking to such Third-Party Sites via the QR Codes does not imply an endorsement or sponsorship of such Third-Party Sites or the information, products, or services offered on or through the Third-Party Sites, nor does it imply an endorsement or sponsorship of this publication by the owners of such Third-Party Sites.

CONTENTS

Chapter 1: Connecting Fitness and Nutrition	7
Chapter 2: How Calories Work	19
Chapter 3: All About Carbs	31
Chapter 4: All About Protein	43
Chapter 5: All About Fat	57
Chapter 6: Hydration	69
Chapter 7: Balancing Your Diet	79
Series Glossary of Key Terms	92
Further Reading & Internet Resources	93
Index	94
Author Biography, Photo Credits & Educational Video Links	96

KEY ICONS TO LOOK FOR

WORDS TO UNDERSTAND: These words, with their easy-to-understand definitions, will increase readers' understanding of the text while building vocabulary skills.

SIDEBARS: This boxed material within the main text allows readers to build knowledge, gain insights, explore possibilities, and broaden their perspectives by weaving together additional information to provide realistic and holistic perspectives.

EDUCATIONAL VIDEOS: Readers can view videos by scanning our QR codes, providing them with additional educational content to supplement the text.

TEXT-DEPENDENT QUESTIONS: These questions send the reader back to the text for more careful attention to the evidence presented there.

RESEARCH PROJECTS: Readers are pointed toward areas of further inquiry connected to each chapter. Suggestions are provided for projects that encourage deeper research and analysis.

SERIES GLOSSARY OF KEY TERMS: This back-of-the-book glossary contains terminology used throughout this series. Words found here increase the reader's ability to read and comprehend higher-level books and articles in this field.

WORDS TO UNDERSTAND

atrophy—the wasting away of body tissue or an organ
eustress—moderate or normal physiological stress that is beneficial for the experiencer
homeostasis—the state of equilibrium between two or more elements, especially within the human body

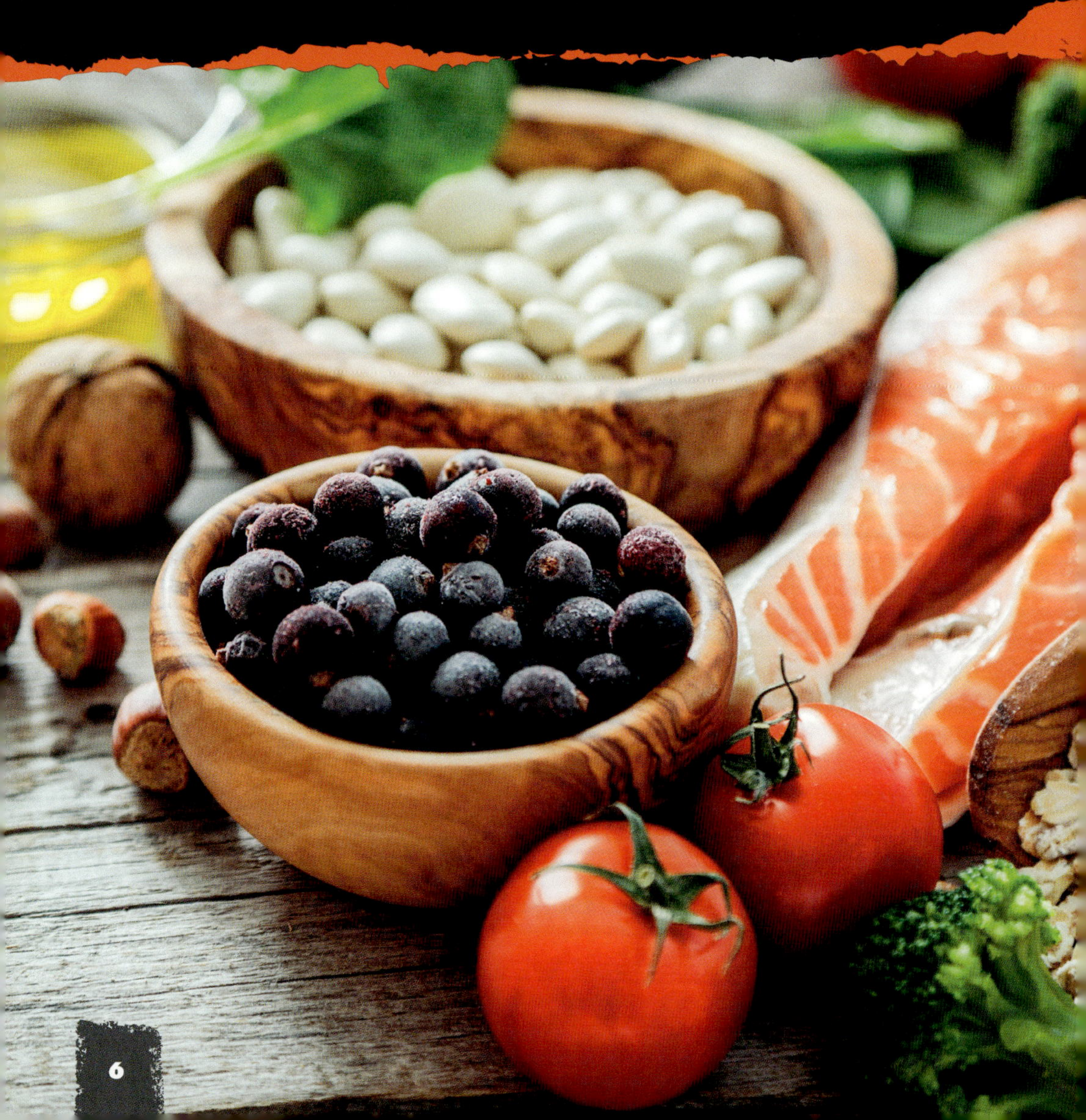

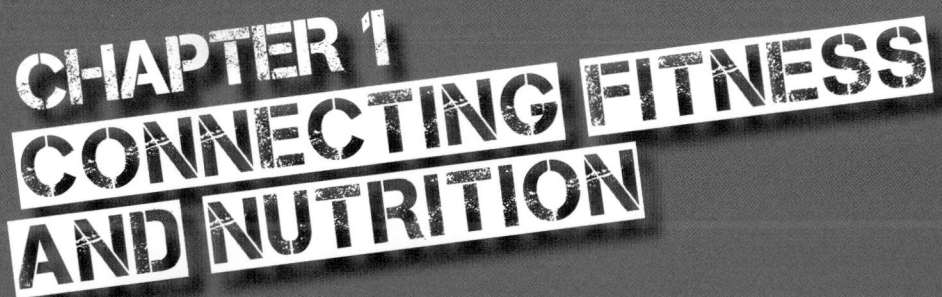

CHAPTER 1
CONNECTING FITNESS AND NUTRITION

FITNESS VS. HEALTH— WHAT'S THE DIFFERENCE?

Fitness, nutrition, and health all exist in a similar space. They all impact the human body, and being vigilant about all three is generally considered to be good for you. Is there a difference between being healthy and being fit? How does nutrition play a role in all of it? Let's attempt to answer these questions.

Let's start with health. Technically, health is defined as "the condition of being sound in body, mind, or spirit; especially: freedom from physical disease or pain." Feeling sick or rundown has an impact on our overall health. The same goes for being emotionally stressed, malnourished, or physically unfit. Fitness and nutrition, therefore, are both things that can *impact* our health.

You may have heard the saying, "You are what you eat." In many cases, that's true. Your cells are constantly growing, dying, reproducing, and otherwise changing in response to their environment. Part of that environment comes from food and water. Your diet quite literally provides the nutrients to build cellular structures, as well as signal storage, transformation, and distribution of information.

Exercise has a similar impact. Assuming you don't overexert yourself too often, exercise is considered **eustress**. As the opposite of distress, eustress refers to moderate or normal physiological stress that is beneficial for the experiencer. Running, for example, can seem hard at first, but eventually improves mood, heart health, and metabolism. Basically, exercise is another outside stimulus that alters internal physiology (a.k.a. health).

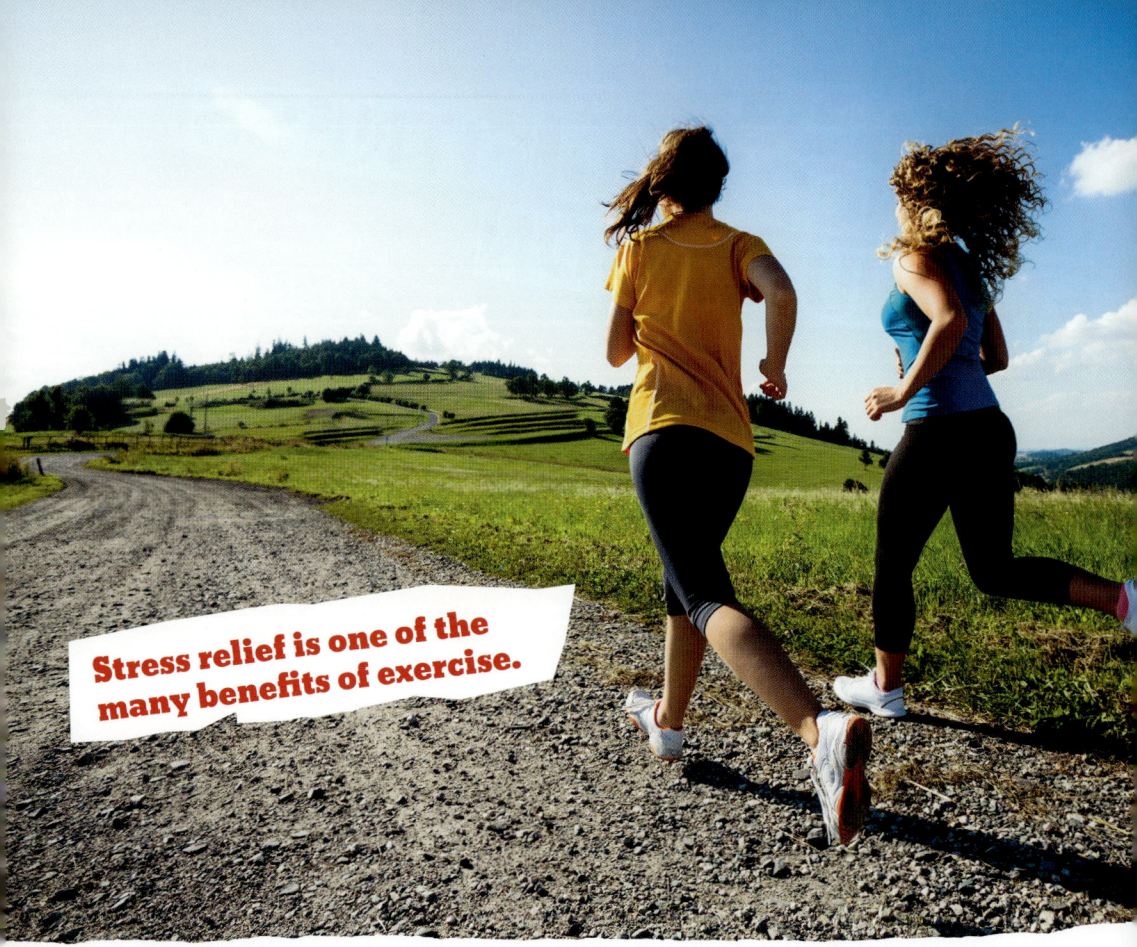

Stress relief is one of the many benefits of exercise.

Fitness, on the other hand, takes a slightly different approach to health. According to the U.S. Department of Health and Human Services, physical fitness is defined as "a set of attributes that people have or achieve that relates to the ability to perform physical activity." Within overall fitness lie different attributes—cardiorespiratory capacity, strength, flexibility, speed and power, endurance, body composition, and more. Someone could be extremely fit, such as a marathon runner, yet be unable to lift anywhere near the same amount of weight as a bodybuilder. Therefore, fitness is a bit trickier to define. Regardless, developing fitness in a specific area will generally improve your overall health.

While it's clear that fitness and nutrition BOTH impact your health, let's take a closer look at the impact they have on each other.

 **Explore the link between food, exercise, and sleep.**

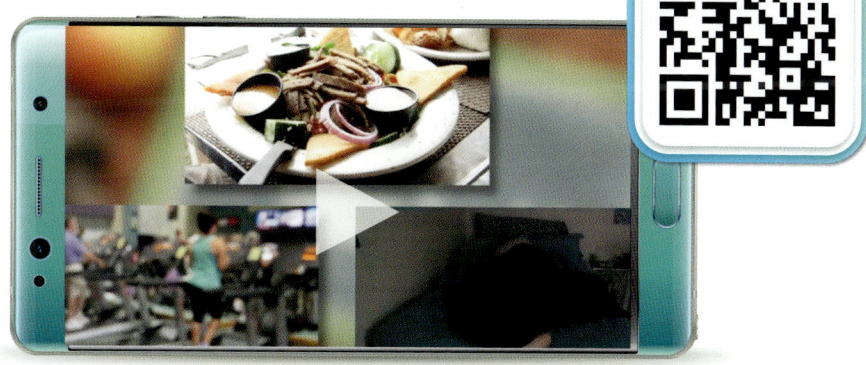

CAN YOU EAT WHATEVER YOU WANT IF YOU EXERCISE?

The short answer is no.

Remember, nutrition directly contributes to your overall health. Food is so much more than calories. It contains the proteins you need to build muscle, the carbohydrates (carbs) you need for energy, or the fats you need to build your cells. It also contains micronutrients—vitamins and minerals that help to start your metabolism or maintain **homeostasis**.

Young people need enough protein to make new tissue, grow bone, and develop hormonally. Moreover, the need for vitamins and minerals increases during adolescence. The more high-quality food you consume, the greater the chance you get the necessary nutrients. According to research, eating any less than 1800 calories per day makes it tough to consume enough vitamin A, copper, vitamin B6, iron, or magnesium.

So, while exercise is healthy, it doesn't automatically negate anything unhealthy you put into your body.

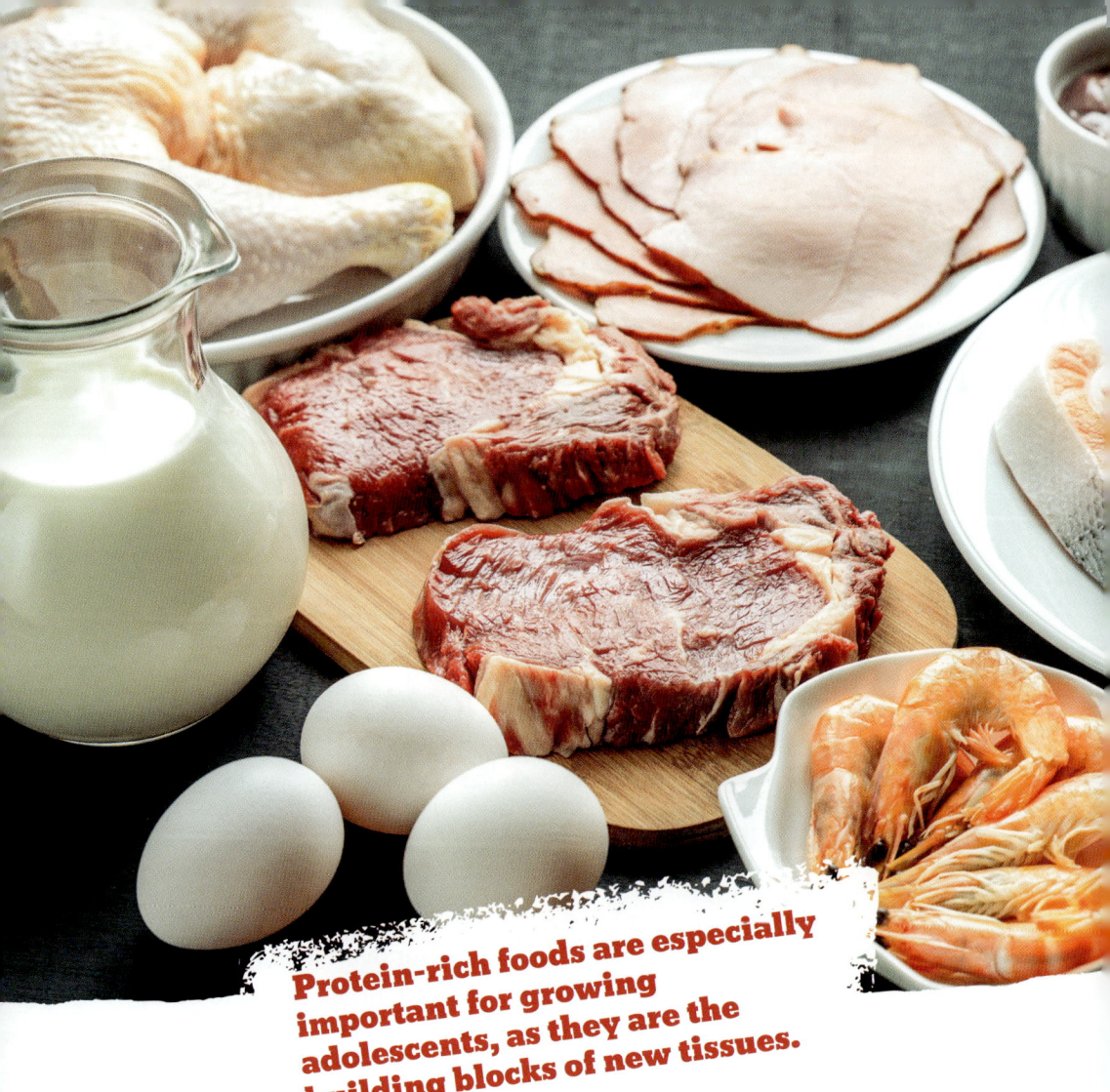

Protein-rich foods are especially important for growing adolescents, as they are the building blocks of new tissues.

Eating things like fast food, processed foods, and too much sugar can still negatively impact your health, even if you exercise. For one, most of those foods are missing important nutrients. Filling up on nutrient-sparse food, even if you eat enough calories, will leave necessary ingredients missing in your diet.

Furthermore, you need fuel in order to exercise! For example, endurance exercise relies on healthy carbs. Muscle-building activities call upon lean proteins, and recovering from intense exercise requires healthy fats. Eating a bunch of junk food doesn't exactly fuel your performance.

CAN YOU BE CONSIDERED FIT IF YOU EAT A HEALTHY, BALANCED DIET BUT DON'T EXERCISE?

If diet is so important to health, where does that leave exercise? Do you have to exercise as long as you're eating the proper nutrients?

In the short term, you can survive without exercise. In the long term, you'll want *some* form of regular movement to thrive. Inactivity is known to decrease circulation, reduce muscular strength and tone, decrease bone density, increase inflammation, and disrupt your immune system function. Not exercising, therefore, elevates your risk of developing the following:

- Cancer
- Stroke
- Type 2 diabetes
- Heart disease
- High blood pressure

THE TRUE CONSEQUENCES OF NOT EATING WELL

In 2019, CNN reported a case study about a young boy who succumbed to blindness as a result of his diet. Apparently, he survived on a diet of french fries, white bread, and Pringles... until his health began to decline. At just fourteen years of age, the University of Bristol began caring for him as he complained of extreme fatigue despite normal BMI, height, and other health indicators. According to the *Annals of Internal Medicine*, medical professionals discovered dangerously low levels of vitamin B12 and red blood cells. Despite receiving treatment, the boy began to lose his hearing and vision within a year. He was blind by the age of seventeen as a result of high zinc levels, as well as low copper, selenium, vitamin D, and vitamin B12. Even if he didn't show any outward signs of malnutrition, clearly not eating well had its negative effects.

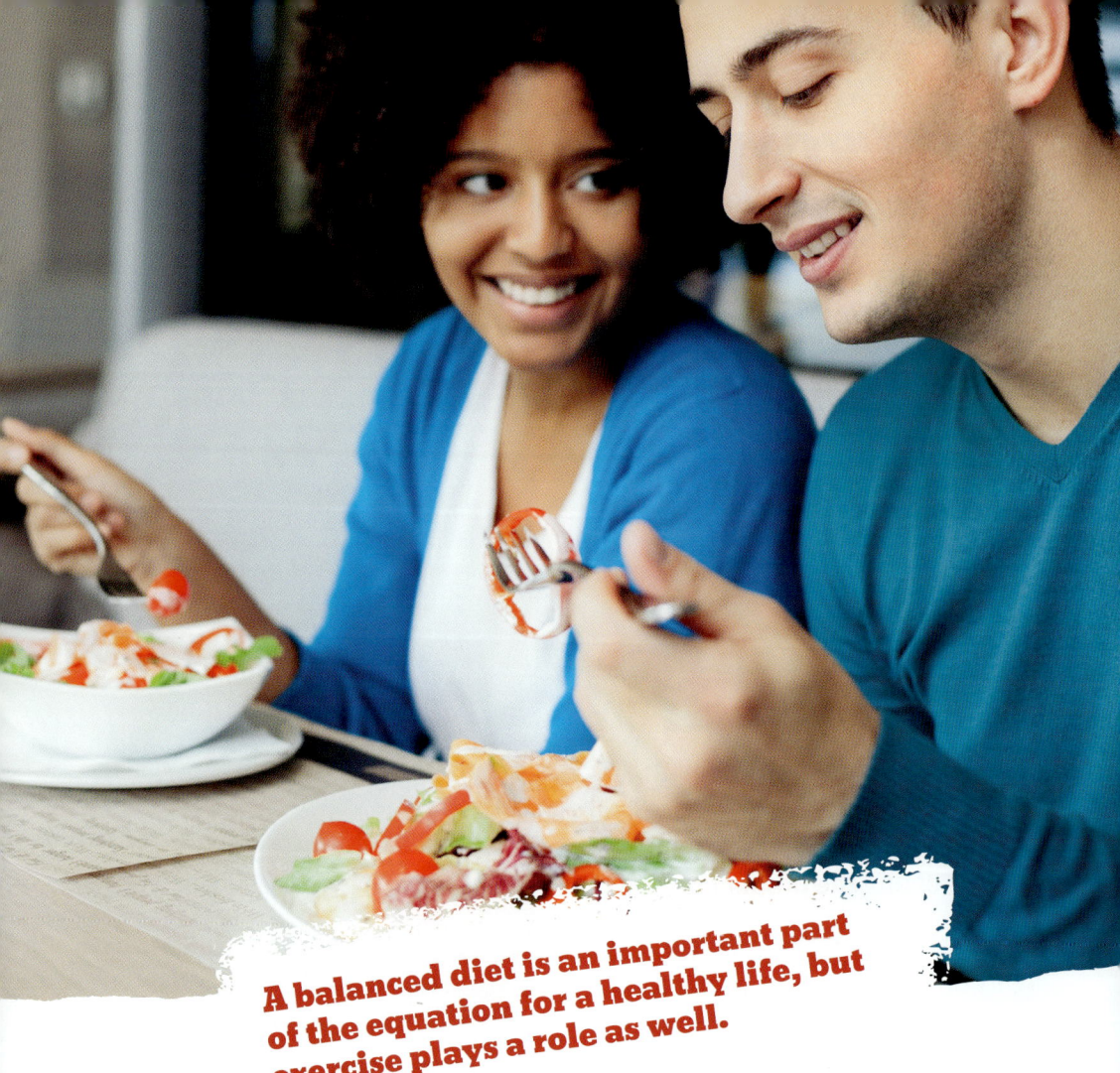

A balanced diet is an important part of the equation for a healthy life, but exercise plays a role as well.

To further illuminate the importance of movement, let's look at the most severe cases of an exercise-free life—being bedridden. Many people suffer from paralysis, disease, or other conditions that prevent them from leaving their beds. According to *Canadian Family Physician*, complications from being bedridden include:

- Muscular **atrophy**
- Impaired muscle endurance
- Osteoporosis due to lack of bone use
- Degenerative joint disease

- Elevated resting heart rate
- Decreased cardiac reserve
- Venous thromboembolism (dangerous blood clots)

With that being said, the above are symptoms of extreme sedentary lifestyles. No one's saying you have to lift weights every day or run 45 miles a week. Simply moving around, stretching, going for walks, or playing sports regularly is enough.

Remember—there are multiple aspects of fitness. Try and pick something you enjoy doing to stay active. The Department of Health and Human Services recommends 60 minutes per day of daily physical activity, whether it's aerobic, muscle building, or bone strengthening.

WHICH IS MORE ESSENTIAL TO FITNESS—DIET OR EXERCISE?

For true fitness, defined as the ability to complete a physical task, exercise takes a slight lead. On the other hand, one could argue that your diet has a larger impact on health. In reality, they're equally as important.

Let's say you have a specific athletic goal, such as winning the state championship. Training for your sport is *obviously* more important than what you eat. Someone who has an impeccable diet but has never played a sport will usually lose to someone with elite experience (but who enjoys ice cream and pizza every once in a while).

What if you compare two people with the same experience, same work ethic, and the same talent level? Athlete A fuels their training with lean proteins, healthy carbs, and plenty of water. Athlete B drinks lots of pop, continues to rely on fast food, and whatever else they feel like eating.

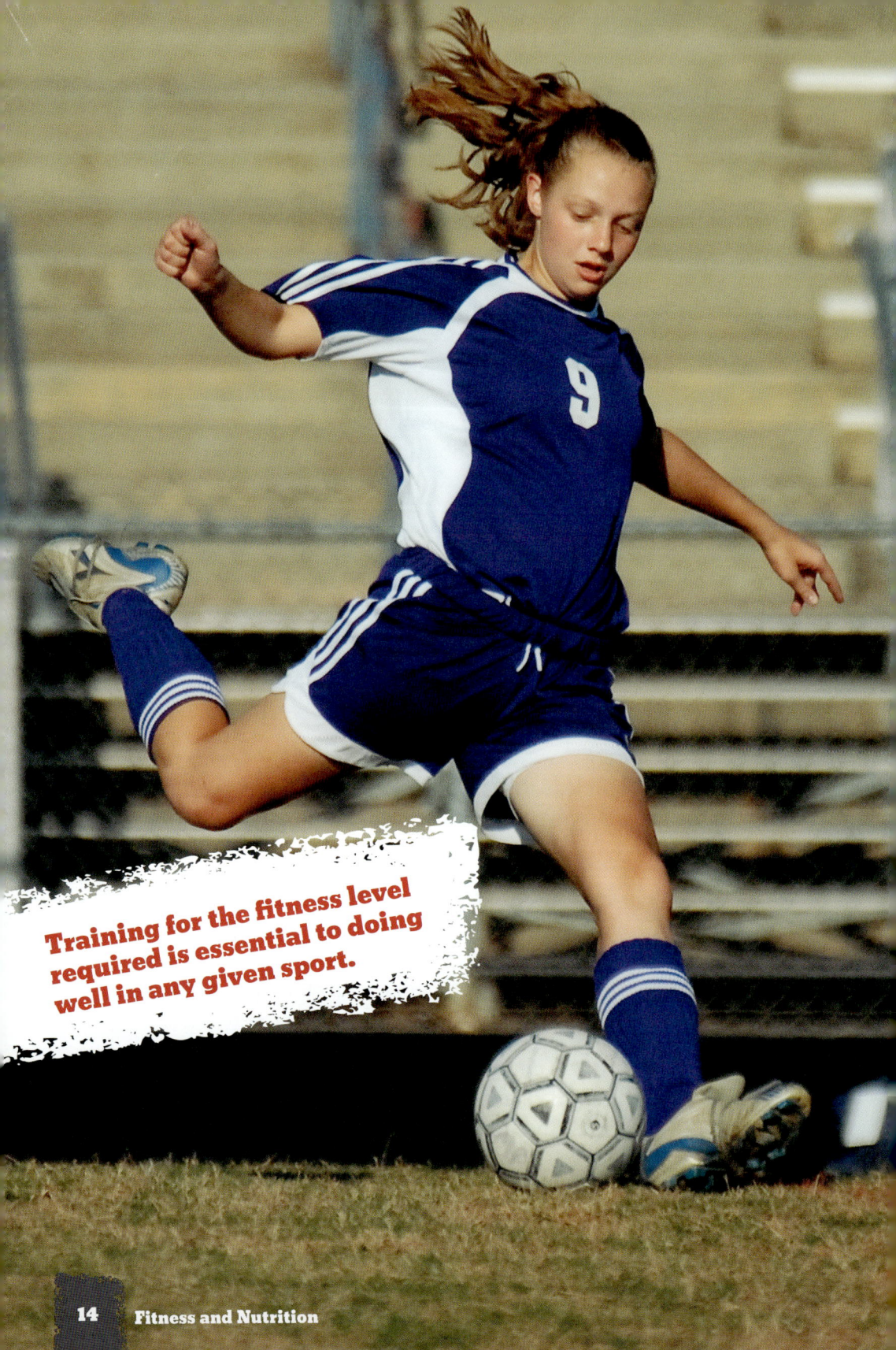

Training for the fitness level required is essential to doing well in any given sport.

Thanks to her nutrition, Athlete A will have more energy at practice. As a result, she'll be able to go farther and faster. She'll recover better after practices and games, and show up the next day energized, ready to train. Her reaction time improves. She gets more out of drills and skills. Athlete A gets 1 percent better every day.

Athlete B, on the other hand, runs out of energy 30 minutes into practice. She has motivation to go farther and faster, but her body is out of fuel. Still, she drains every last piece of energy, becoming exhausted after one tough practice. The next day, her muscles are tired from being overworked. She is one step behind, and her skills start to suffer. Athlete B gets 1 percent worse every day.

Who's going to win the state championship?

Even if you don't have an athletic goal, the same applies to general health and wellness. Those who invest in their bodies will continue to grow and flourish. Those who drain their bodies will feel sluggish, tired, and rundown.

THE BLUE ZONES—THE WORLD'S HEALTHIEST POPULATIONS

During a *National Geographic* expedition, scientists investigated certain places around the world where people consistently have longer, healthier, and happier lives. In fact, people in these places are living to age one hundred at 10 times the normal rate. They dubbed these areas the "Blue Zones," and they can be found in California, Costa Rica, Japan, Italy, and Greece. But what makes these populations so different?

Well, as it turned out, it appears to be due to their way of life. In addition to having a strong purpose, sense of community, and less stress, these uber-healthy people ate well and exercised regularly—

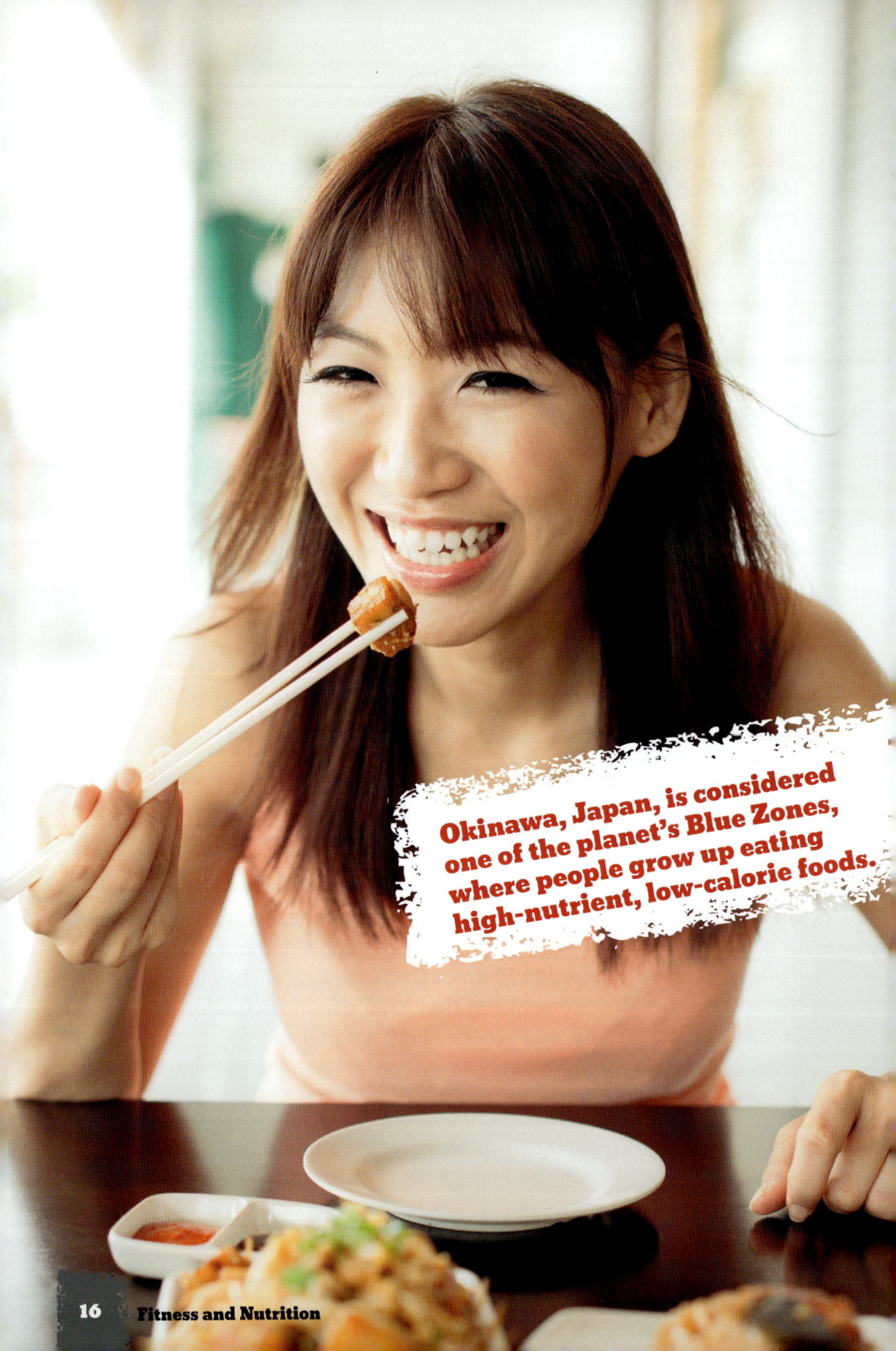
Okinawa, Japan, is considered one of the planet's Blue Zones, where people grow up eating high-nutrient, low-calorie foods.

in a surprisingly simple way. Here are some of the guidelines that researchers discovered:

- Move naturally—those who live the longest don't hit the gym every day or compete in marathons. Instead, they go for walks, garden, and work outside.
- Follow the 80 percent rule—rather than stuff yourself, eat until you feel 80 percent full. That 80 percent is enough to satisfy you and makes for small meals that maintain a healthy weight.
- Plant slant—at the core of the Blue Zone diet are all types of beans, full of fiber, protein, carbs, and micronutrients. They only enjoy meat a few times per month.

As you can see, none of these are hard, fast, complicated rules. They simply enjoy more plants on their plates, get outside and move more, and don't overindulge. Neither fitness nor diet is more important. Rather, the world's healthiest people practice a balance.

TEXT-DEPENDENT QUESTIONS

1. What are the common side effects of a sedentary lifestyle, regardless of nutrition?
2. Describe 3–4 dietary interventions that can improve one's health.
3. How can eating well improve your fitness, and vice versa?

RESEARCH PROJECT

Investigate one of the Blue Zones mentioned in this chapter. Put together a short presentation on their way of life, including environment, activity level, nutritional practices, recreation, and more.

WORDS TO UNDERSTAND

basal metabolic rate—the amount of energy the body uses to keep you alive, measured under strict laboratory control

caloric density—the amount of calories in a food item based on its weight

calorie—a unit used to express the heat output of an organism and the fuel or energy value of food

metabolic equivalent of a task (MET)—the ratio of energy expenditure when performing a task compared to rest, which is measured at 3.5 ml O_2 per kg body weight × min

resting metabolic rate—the amount of energy used by the body at rest, typically taken in "real-life" scenarios, outside of strict laboratory conditions

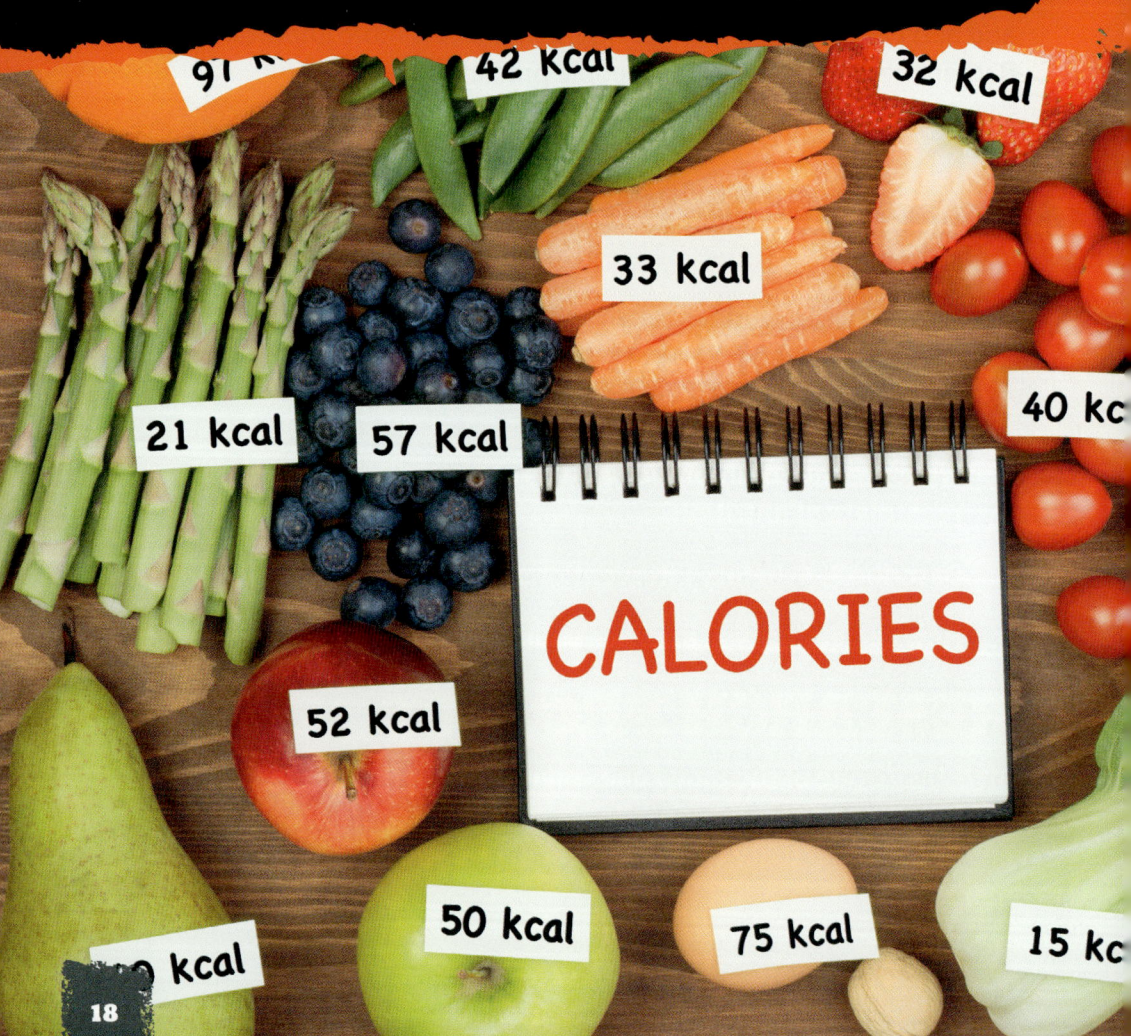

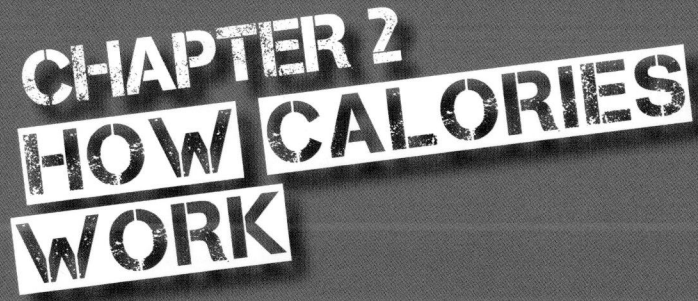

CHAPTER 2
HOW CALORIES WORK

WHAT ARE CALORIES?

Everyone thinks of **calories** as this abstract concept entangled with what we eat. We consume so many calories each day as well as burn them through movement and exercise. But what is a calorie?

Simply put, a calorie is a unit of energy. It has the same value as 4.186 joules and could be produced by your car, coal, or nuclear energy. However, its most common application comes in food.

Ironically, when written in uppercase, a Calorie refers to a kilocalorie, or 4.186 kilojoules of energy. You might not think this matters, but the majority of food labels, internet resources, and books mistakenly write calorie when they really mean *kilo*calorie.

For simplicity, we will continue to use the lowercase "calorie" in reference to kilocalorie, as that is how it is commonly used.

Now that we've gotten that out of the way, calories simply measure how much energy we expend or consume. We need calories to fuel all human activity, from sleeping and breathing to working out.

MEASURING CALORIES IN YOUR DIET

Everything you eat (assuming it's an actual food) has caloric value. The tissues within plants, meats, or fats store calories for later use. When you eat, your body consumes them, breaks them down, and utilizes that stored energy for its own benefit.

You might think that the more you eat, the more calories you consume. Sometimes that's true. Sometimes it isn't.

 What is a calorie? Watch this to learn more about this energy unit.

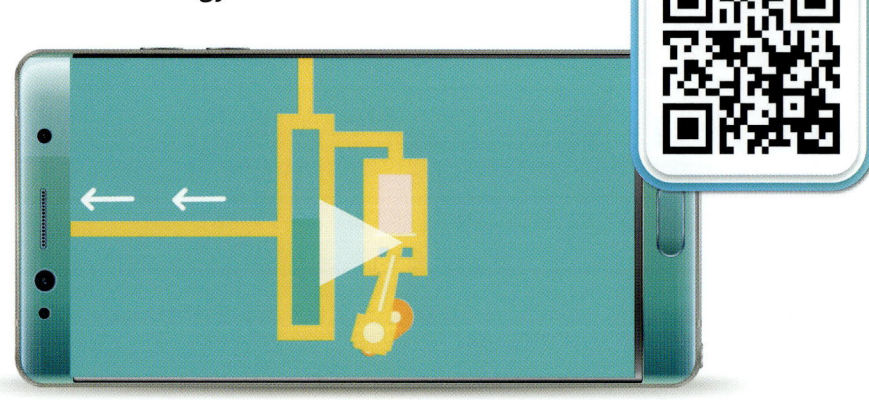

Keeping track of the actual number of calories consumed is a tricky task. Tracking caloric density is a more reliable method for the calorie-conscious.

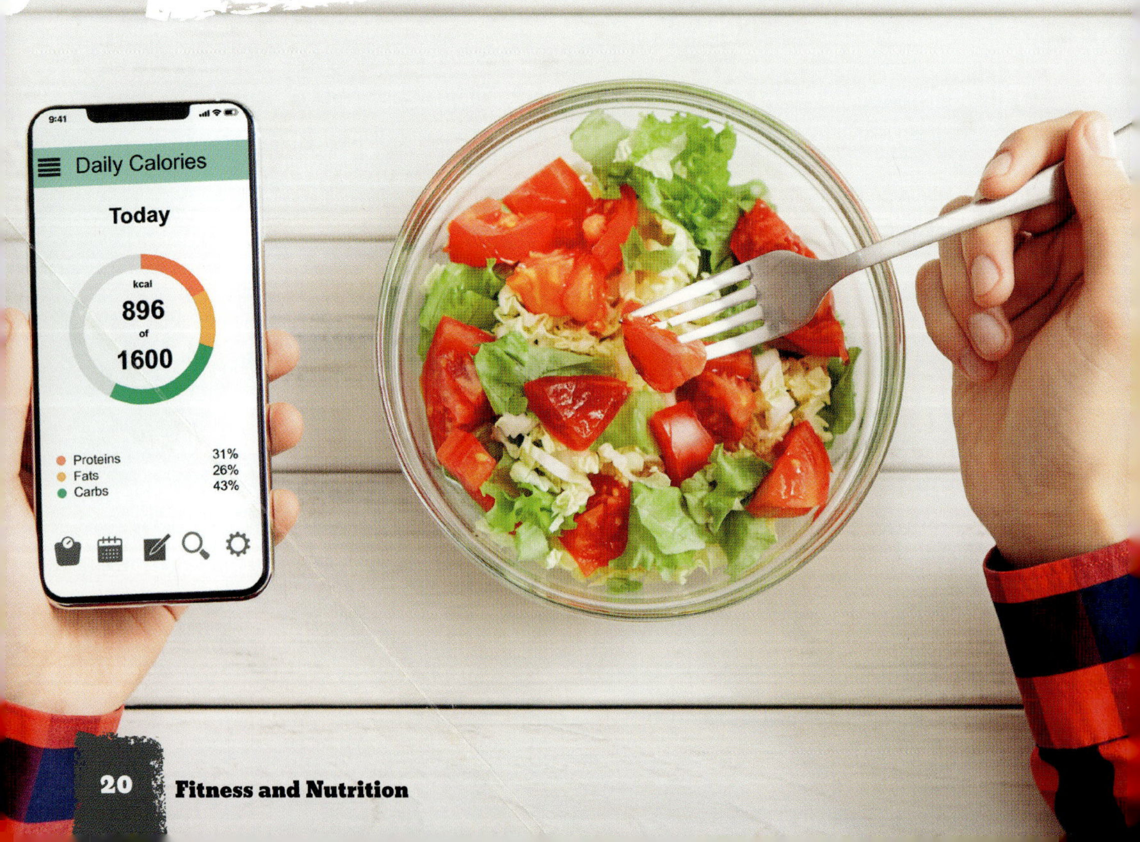

Fitness and Nutrition

Caloric density

Calorie counting is a complex process that can differ based on labeling, method of cooking, absorption, or a myriad of other factors. However, it's pretty easy to discern the caloric density of a food. **Caloric density** refers to the amount of calories in a food item based on weight. For example, a bag of potato chips weighs next to nothing but can leave you consuming hundreds of calories. For the same amount of calories, you could eat an entire bunch of broccoli, which weighs in significantly heavier. The broccoli, therefore, has a low caloric density (low calories per weight), whereas the chips have a high caloric density (high amount of calories per weight).

Why this matters

If we were starving, we'd want foods with the least caloric density—that is to say, the maximum amount of energy for the least amount of food. However, in North America, most of us aren't starving. We generally have access to three square meals per day and aren't hunting down prey to eat every night. Therefore, a lot of people eat highly calorie-dense foods such as fast food, fried foods, and cupcakes, which adversely impacts their health. Eating these foods means we can meet our calorie requirements in one meal. Then they eat lunch and dinner, adding more, unnecessary calories. After weeks and months of eating this way, the body doesn't know what to do with the extra energy. It, therefore, saves it up for some future food-deficient apocalypse, and stores it all away as fat.

Daily calorie requirements

According to Health.gov, daily caloric "estimates range from 1,600 to 2,400 calories per day for adult women and 2,000 to 3,000 calories per day for adult men. Within each age and sex category, the low end of the range is for sedentary individuals; the high end of the range is for active individuals."

For adolescents, however, the requirements tend to be even higher. Teenagers need to fuel their growth and, therefore, need an average of 2,800 calories (boys) or 2,200 calories (girls) per day.

However, these requirements vary depending on your daily activity. For example, an elite cross-country runner needs more fuel than your average high school-aged person.

If you are sedentary (little or no exercise):
calorie calculation = BMR × 1.2

If you are lightly active (light exercise/sports 1–3 days per week):
calorie calculation = BMR × 1.375

If you are moderately active (moderate exercise/sports 3–5 days per week):
calorie calculation = BMR × 1.55

If you are very active (hard exercise/sports 6–7 days a week):
calorie calculation = BMR × 1.725

If you are extra active (very hard exercise/sports and physical job or 2x training):
calorie calculation = BMR × 1.9

BURNING CALORIES

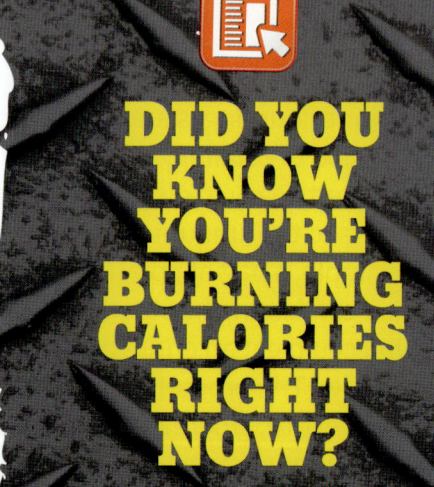

DID YOU KNOW YOU'RE BURNING CALORIES RIGHT NOW?

By simply existing, your body works to circulate blood, digest food, fuel brain activity, and more. These processes require energy. To create energy, we rely on metabolism. Specifically, our bodies refer to mitochondria. Small organelles within your cells, mitochondria are the powerhouses of the body. They transform nutrients and calories into usable energy. They're constantly working to keep you going. So, the more demands you place on your body, the more energy they have to produce.

Burning calories is a hot topic, but it doesn't require much effort, as the body needs calories to survive. Your **basal metabolic rate** (BMR) refers to the amount of energy the body uses to keep you alive. No digestion, no texting on your phone, nothing else. You can think of this as the energy output required to sleep. It's typically measured in a lab using complex equipment.

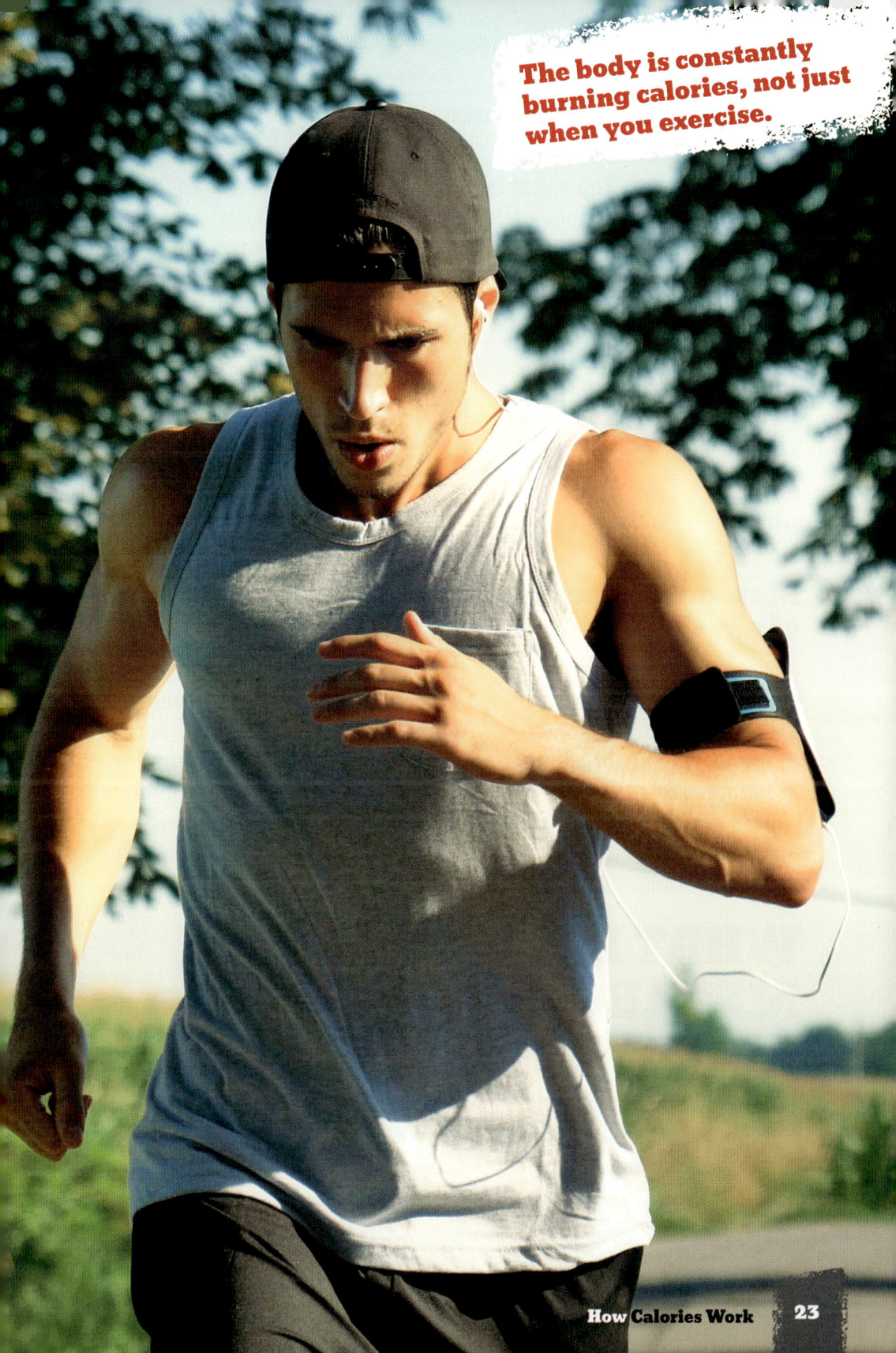

The body is constantly burning calories, not just when you exercise.

Resting metabolic rate

Resting metabolic rate (RMR), on the other hand, refers to the amount of energy you use at rest. This term is used interchangeably with BMR, but technically BMR requires you to be reclined, fasted, and in a laboratory setting. RMR is a more realistic measure of everyday life.

Adult Male:

$$RMR = 88.362 + (13.397 \times \text{weight in kg}) + (4.799 \times \text{height in cm}) - (5.677 \times \text{age in years})$$

Adult Female:

$$RMR = 447.593 + (9.247 \times \text{weight in kg}) + (3.098 \times \text{height in cm}) - (4.330 \times \text{age in years})$$

Metabolic equivalent of a task

Metabolic equivalent of a task (MET) refers to how much energy your body will need to produce to complete it successfully. Your RMR equals one MET, and everything else refers back to that. For example, walking briskly averages at around 4 METs, while running at 10 mph takes 16 METs. However, age, fitness level, and task-related experience come into play. For example, it takes a lot less energy for swimming great Michael Phelps to swim one lap than it does the average person.

WHAT ELSE AFFECTS METABOLISM AND CALORIE BURN?

Ultimately, multiple factors play into calorie burn. One obvious element is exercise. Work harder, expend more energy, and burn more calories. Yet we often neglect the other factors, such as muscle mass, age, gut health, and hormonal profile.

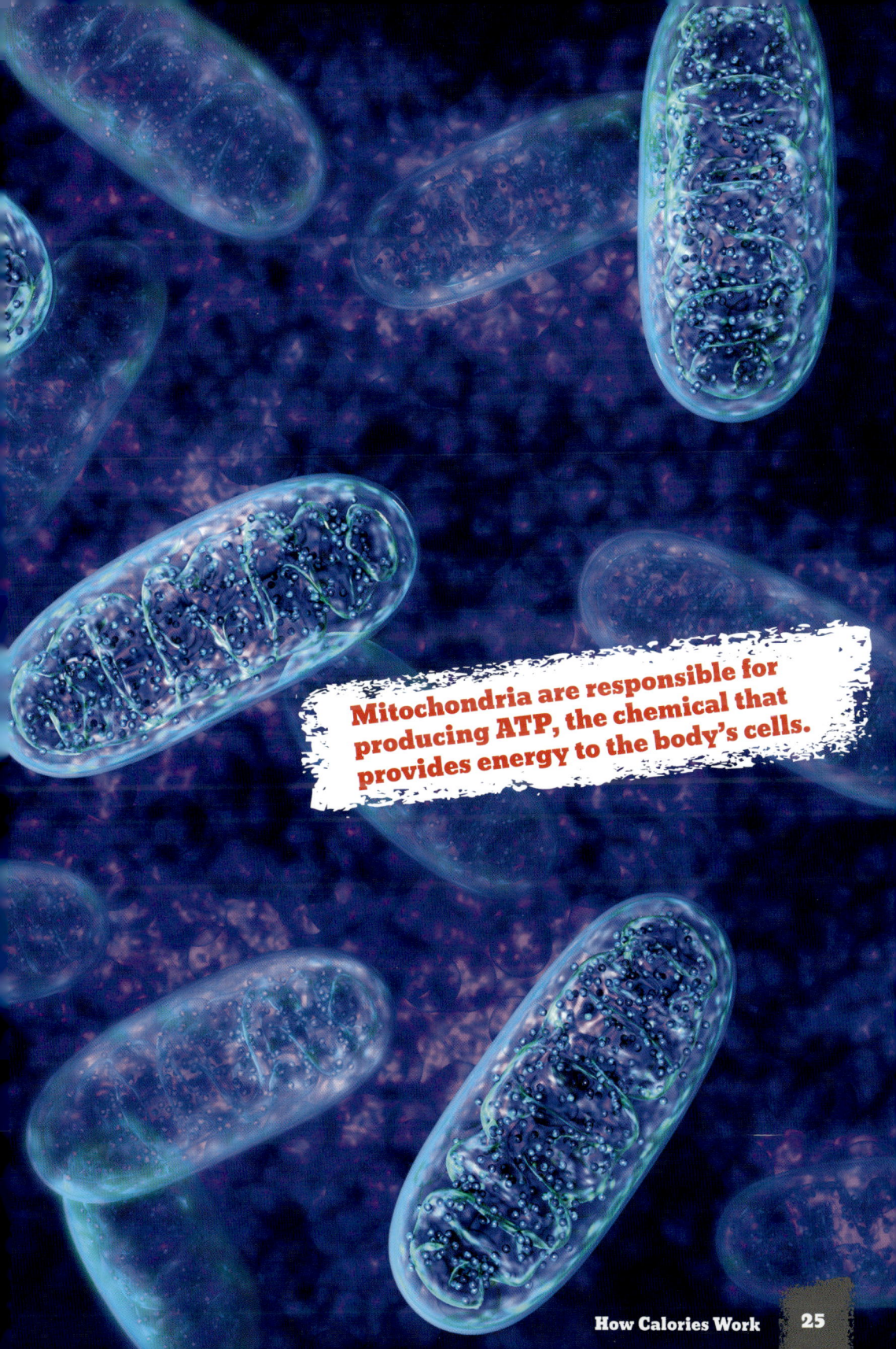

Mitochondria are responsible for producing ATP, the chemical that provides energy to the body's cells.

How Calories Work

Lean muscle mass

By simply sitting on your body, your muscles are burning energy. In fact, they're the most metabolically active tissue in the body. That's because that's where your energy-burning organelles, the mitochondria, live. The amount of calories muscles burn at rest varies based on mitochondrial density and total muscle mass. Despite these variations, experts agree that skeletal muscle mass largely affects total resting energy expenditure, and likely enhances your capabilities to work harder in the gym. As such, those looking to improve their metabolic rate should first aim to add muscle.

Age

As we grow older, our metabolism matures as well. Our BMR declines with age. While infants obviously require less energy than active teenagers (simply due to size alone), the rate of metabolism starts to gradually decrease in adults. Experts relate this fact to loss of muscle mass, fat tissue, and physical activity. However, if energy intake exceeds the decreased need, abdominal fat can start to accumulate and reduce glucose tolerance, leading to other health issues. Therefore, staying physically active can offset changes in metabolism.

Hormones

Testosterone, for example, plays a pivotal role in carb, fat, and protein metabolism. It also regulates growth hormone, which can turn food into muscle mass. Studies showed that testosterone deficiency is associated with decreased glucose tolerance, increased body fat, and higher cholesterol levels.

Another metabolic hormone, insulin, can disrupt your calorie burn if your body is sensitive to it. If your body doesn't respond to insulin as it should, your blood sugar stays elevated. Excess sugar needs somewhere to go, however, so it gets stored as fat. Then, when it's actually time to burn calories, your body won't need to reach into fat stores. As a result, you can end up with metabolic syndrome, or dysfunction of the body's ability to burn calories properly.

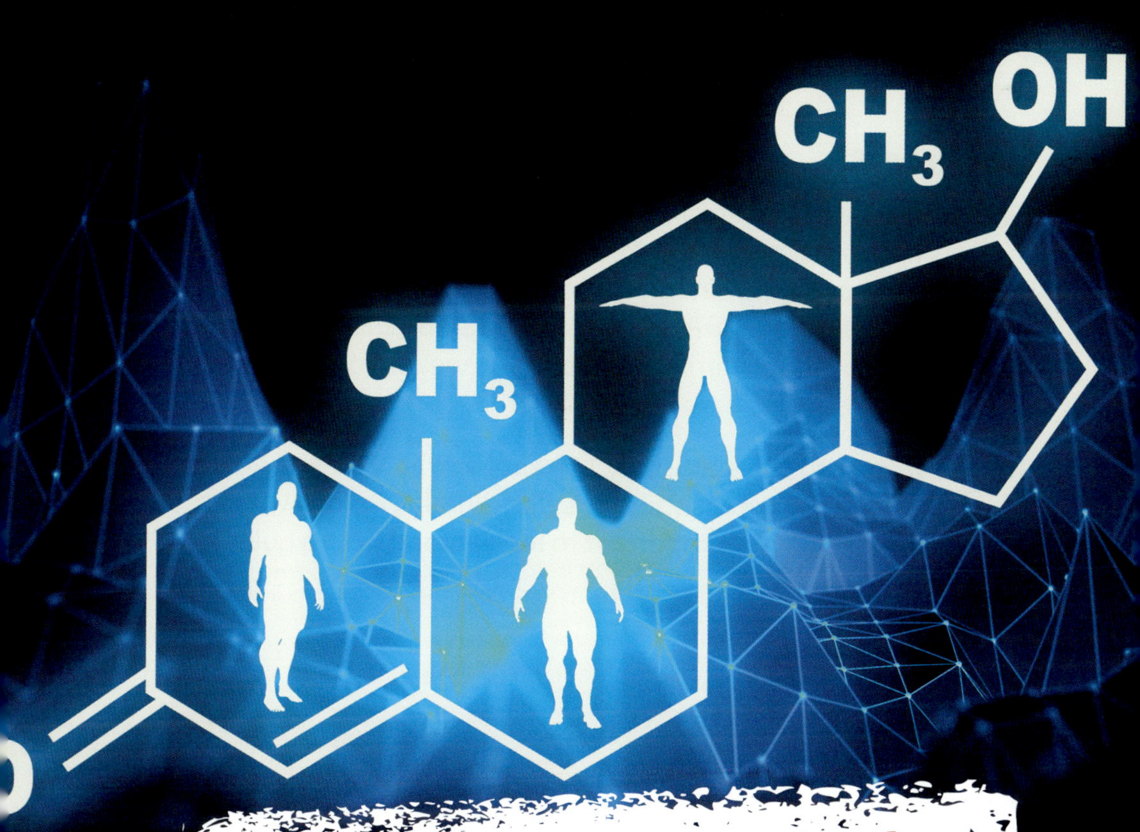

Testosterone, a hormone made up of carbon, hydrogen, and oxygen (C19H28O2), helps the body regulate things such as body fat and cholesterol levels.

Insulin and its role in the human body is explained in this short video.

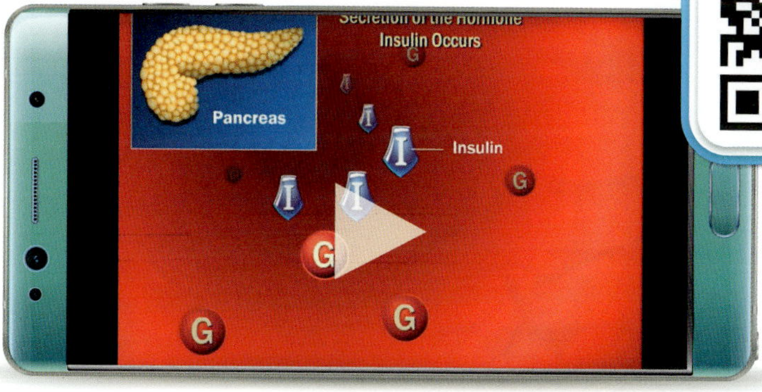

How Calories Work

Gut health

Finally, the overall gut environment can affect how you metabolize food. As food passes through the digestive system first, those with a normally functioning gut microbiome have a better chance of absorbing usable energy. For example, one study showed a diverse environment of gut bacteria correlates with weight loss, while another showed more efficient carb metabolism.

The above goes to show that diet, metabolism, and general health depend on much more than simple caloric intake. Rather, with so many factors at play, it's important to look at food from a holistic perspective.

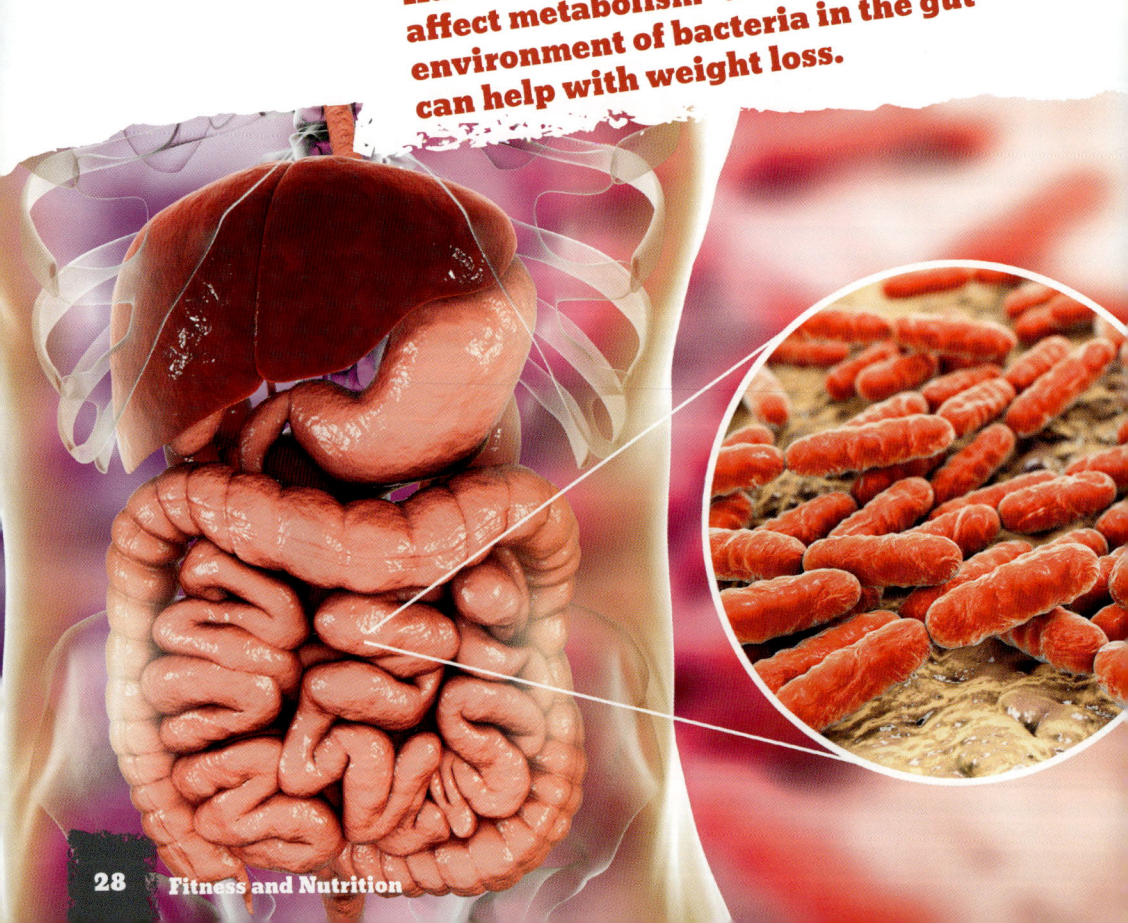

Having a healthy gut can positively affect metabolism—a diverse environment of bacteria in the gut can help with weight loss.

 To maintain a healthy gut, these 10 foods are recommended.

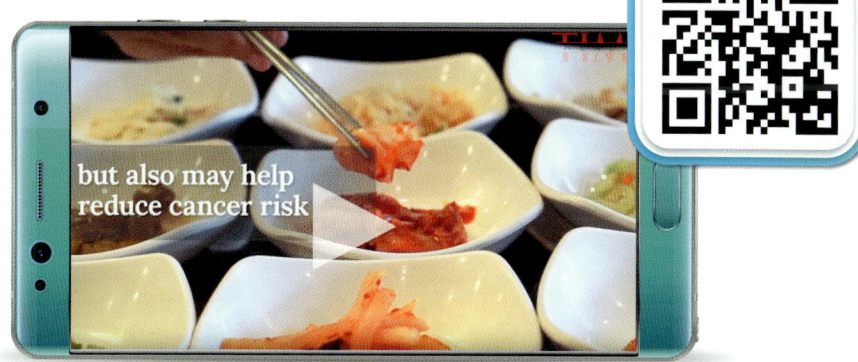

TEXT-DEPENDENT QUESTIONS

1. What is a calorie, and how do humans use it to power activity?

2. Name at least three factors that go into your daily caloric requirement, and why it varies from person to person.

3. What is a food's caloric density, and how might it affect your meal choices?

RESEARCH PROJECT

Michael Phelps turned heads when he reportedly ate a diet of 12,000 calories per day in preparation for the Beijing Olympics. While this may have been a myth or exaggeration, research the metabolic demands of competing in various sports. Pick an athlete and study his or her average daily practice times, energy output, and lean muscle mass. How might an Olympian's diet, for example, change to meet his or her demands during preparation? How would his or her muscle mass affect the athlete's RMR on non-training days? Present your answers in a two-page report.

How Calories Work 29

WORDS TO UNDERSTAND

disaccharide—a compound formed by the union of two monosaccharides
glycemic index—a carbohydrate's rate of digestion and effect on blood sugar, relative to glucose
glycolysis—the first step in the metabolic breakdown of glucose
ketosis—a process through which the liver produces ketone bodies for fuel
monosaccharide—the most basic form of a sugar

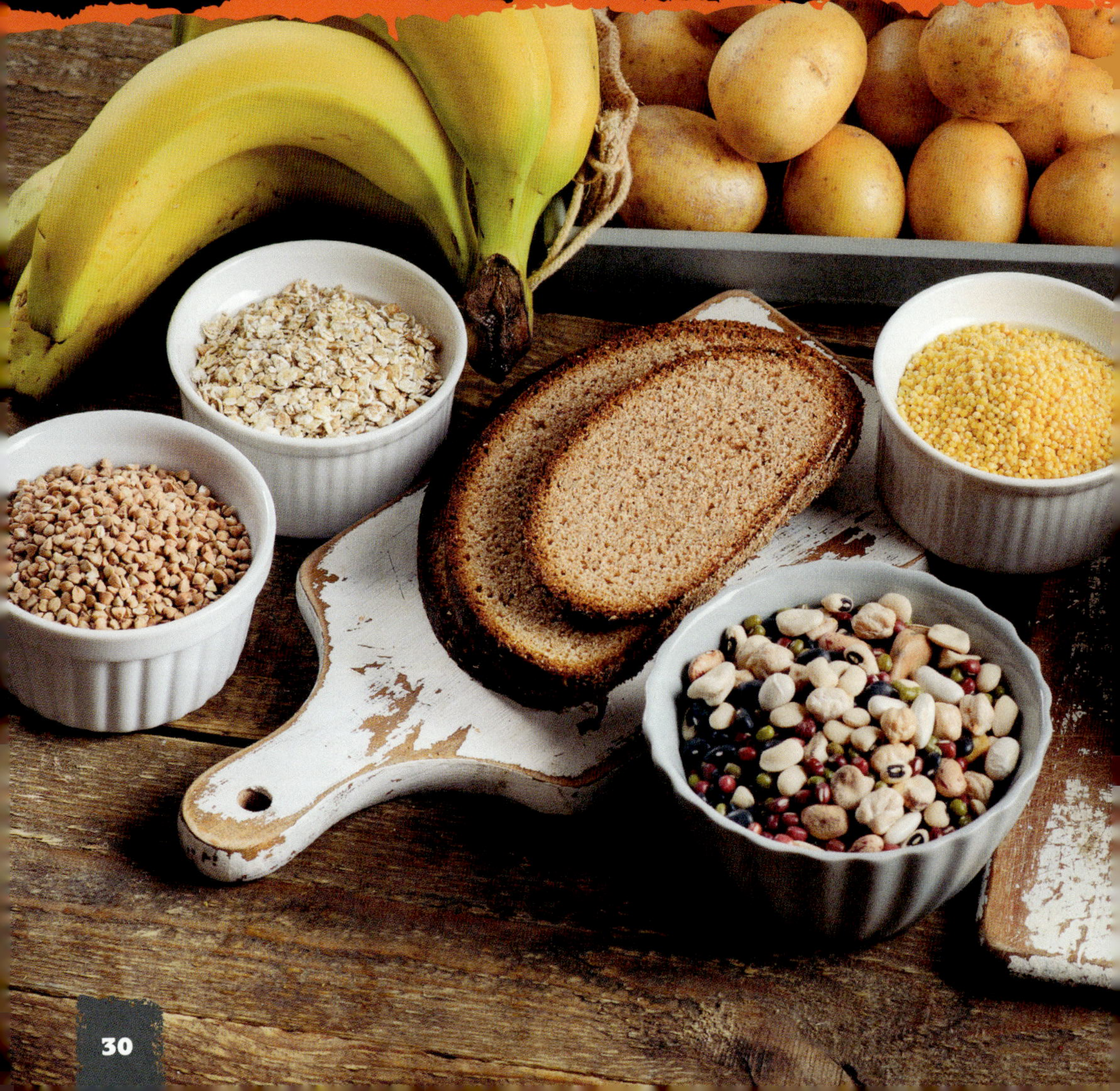

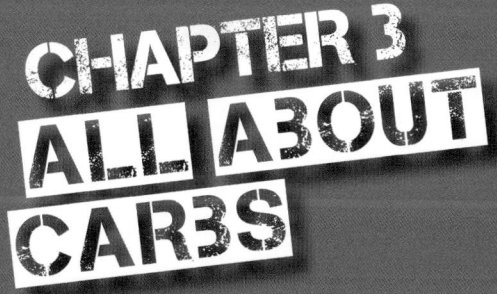

CHAPTER 3
ALL ABOUT CARBS

WHAT DEFINES A CARB?

Carbohydrates are one of the four macronutrients. As such, they are critical to human function, specifically energy production, breaking down fatty acids, regulating blood sugar, and cognition.

Dietary carbs fall into two basic categories—simple and complex.

Also known as simple sugars and starches, these two variations of carbs differ in their chemical nature. The fewer saccharide chains involved, the less complex the carb. At their most basic, called **monosaccharides**, carbs come in one of three forms—glucose, fructose, or galactose. These all combine in some way, shape, or form to create other carbs.

For example, the **disaccharides** are either lactose (glucose + galactose), sucrose (glucose + fructose), or maltose (glucose + glucose). Despite being slightly more complex, these carbs are still considered "simple," meaning the human body rapidly absorbs them.

Complex carbs, on the other hand, consist of polysaccharides. Glycogen and other starches feature multiple chains of these simple sugars, and, therefore, it takes the body longer to break them down.

Benefits of carbs

- Quick energy source (simple carbs)
- Cortisol control post-workout (simple carbs)
- Muscle preservation and recovery (both depending on timing)
- Sustained energy (complex carbs)
- Dietary fiber to aid digestion (complex carbs)

 You've probably heard of carbs, but they aren't all the same. Watch this video to learn the difference.

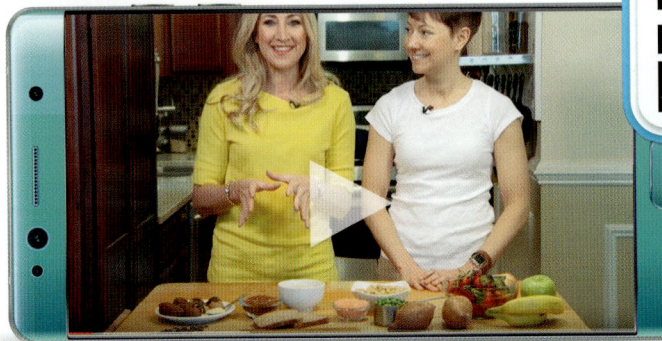

When broken down into glucose, these carbs can be converted into adenosine triphosphate (ATP), or the molecules that give us energy. We can also get ATP from fats or proteins, but glucose is the body's preferred source. Carb supplements, therefore, have the most important nutrient to fuel exercise and recovery.

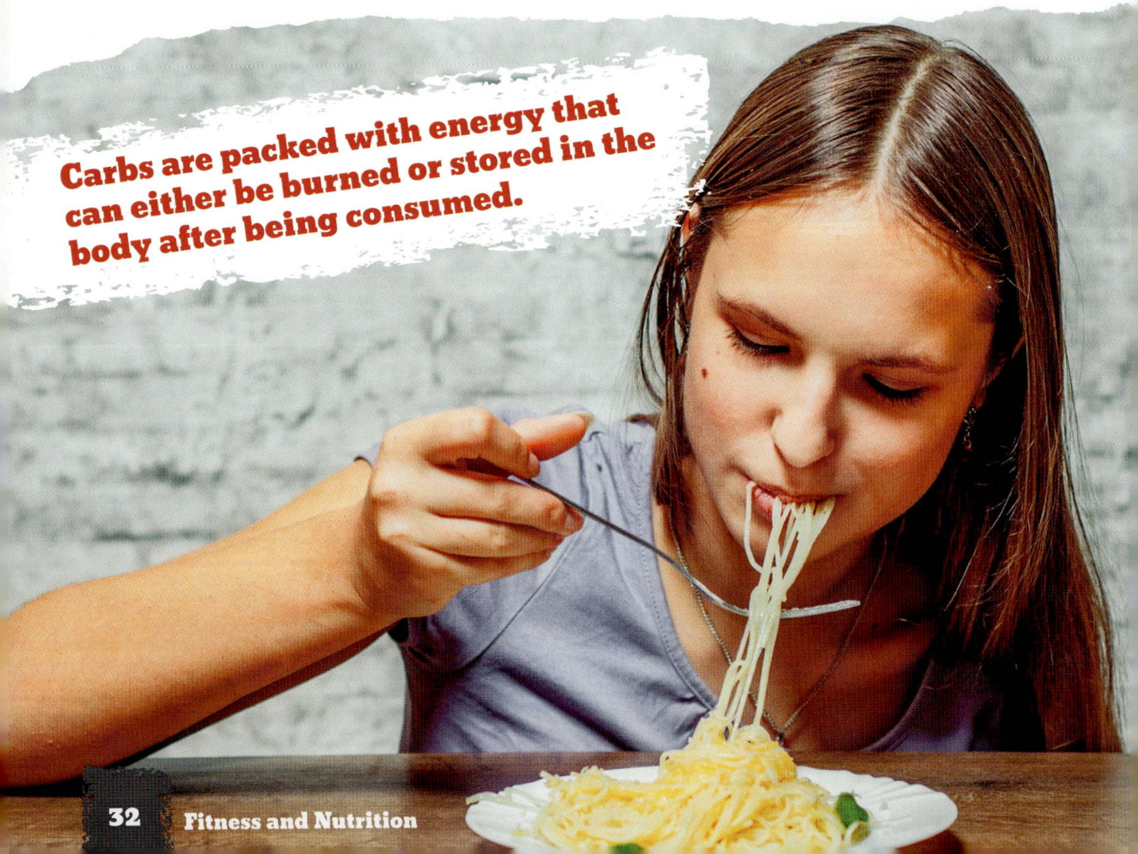

Carbs are packed with energy that can either be burned or stored in the body after being consumed.

WHAT'S WITH ALL THE HYPE?

It seems like you can't turn a corner nowadays without someone villainizing carbs. But where did all of that hype come from?

A part of it has to do with very real health concerns. Consuming simple sugars can elevate your blood sugar and create spikes in a hormone called insulin. In the short term, this provides usable energy for running, working out, or even a really difficult exam. If that energy isn't needed, however, it's transformed into fats for storage, potentially adding to your body fat. Moreover, your cells will learn these insulin spikes aren't doing anything for them. It's sort of like the story of *The Boy Who Cried Wolf*. Your cells will stop believing the signals, and you can develop something called insulin resistance. Insulin resistance is associated with obesity, type II diabetes, and a whole host of health concerns.

Thanks to something called the **glycemic index**, you can determine the impact a carb will have on your body. In short, the glycemic index refers to a carbohydrate's rate of digestion and effect on blood sugar. Glucose (which is blood sugar) is the body's preferred energy source and, therefore, has a glycemic index of 1. All other carbs are measured accordingly. The more complex a carb, the longer it takes to digest, and the less it spikes your insulin levels.

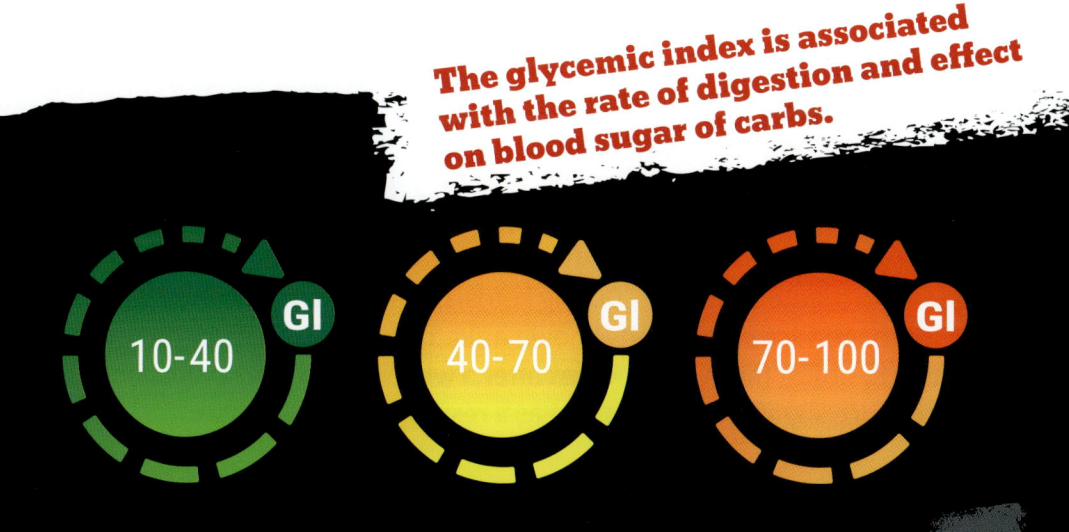

The glycemic index is associated with the rate of digestion and effect on blood sugar of carbs.

10-40 GI   40-70 GI   70-100 GI

All About Carbs

Not all carbs are "bad." In fact, even sugar can be useful if eaten before a workout. Regardless, the sugar scare has recently given rise to low-carb diets.

LOW-CARB DIETING

People have been manipulating the way they eat since the dawn of modern agriculture and the abundance of food. Even the ancient Greeks practiced dietary restrictions. A study in France in the early 20th century found that low-calorie diets and fasting reduced seizures. However, as extremely low-calorie diets aren't sustainable in the long term, seizures would return as soon as patients began eating normally again. Therefore, they started utilizing low-carb measures instead.

A 20th-century physician, Dr. Mynie Peterman of the Mayo Clinic, took this idea and revolutionized it into the ketogenic (keto) diet. His diet championed eating tons of fat for your daily calories. The traditional approach suggests a 4:1 ratio of fat to protein and carbs. The idea is that, in the absence of carbs, the body goes into a state of **ketosis**. During ketosis, the liver breaks down fatty acids to produce compounds known as ketone bodies for fuel. The brain learns to utilize these metabolites after a while, and people typically experience significant weight loss as a result.

DR. ATKINS AND THE ATKINS DIET

We can probably trace the modern low-carb craze back to one person—Dr. Robert Atkins. In the early 1970s, Dr. Atkins launched a book on low-carb dieting, claiming that eating very little sugar/carbs and lots of fats/protein yielded health. In the early 2000s, he revitalized this book; it became a *NY Times* bestseller, and the idea of "net carbs" was introduced. Atkins considered the "net carbs" found in food to be those that the body can actually absorb—not including fiber. Therefore, vegetables were highly encouraged and fruit, bread, and sugar were vilified. People lost tons of weight on this diet, but it came with its own health risk. The Atkins diet was associated with high cholesterol and an increased risk of heart disease.

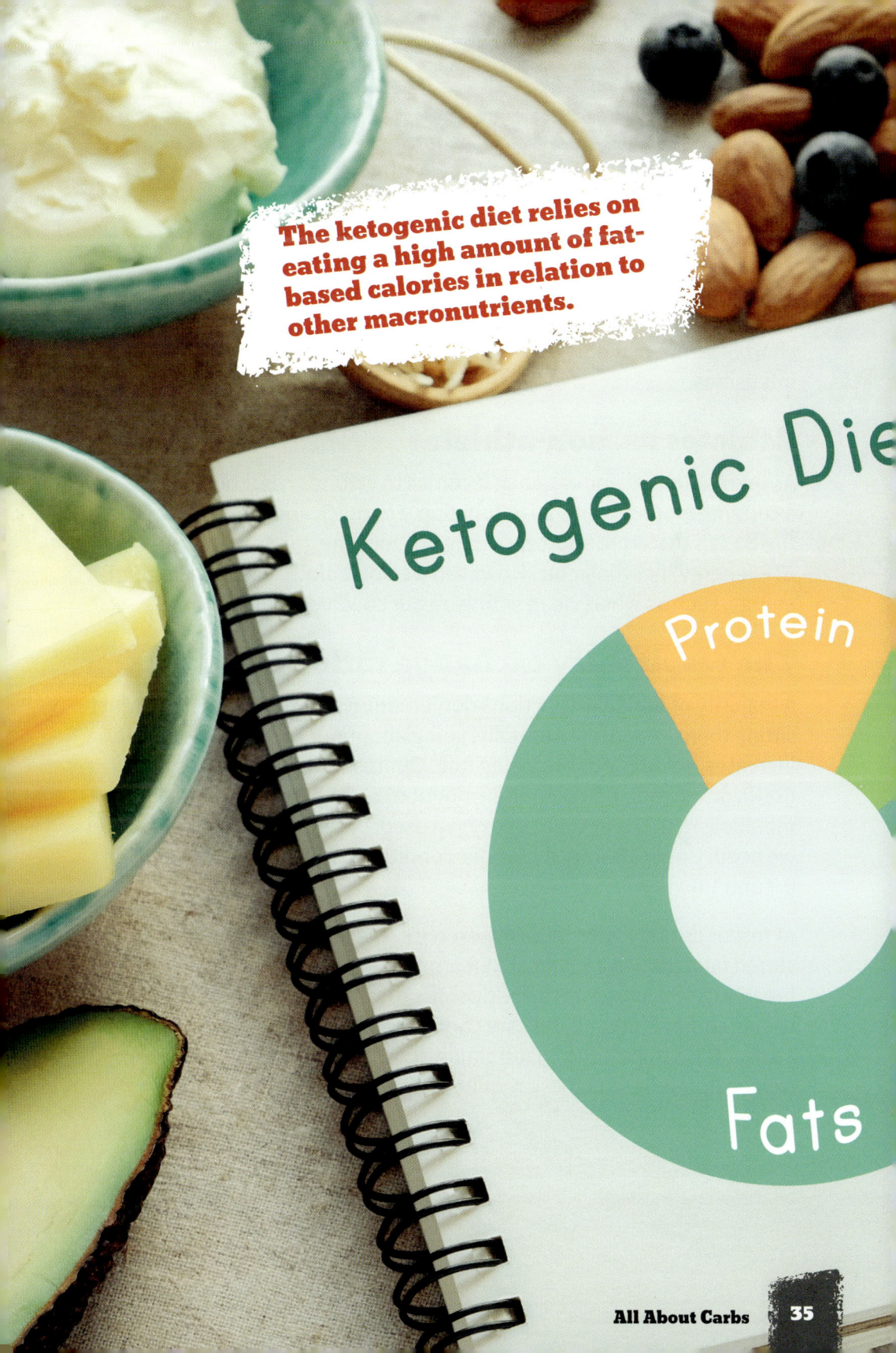

The ketogenic diet relies on eating a high amount of fat-based calories in relation to other macronutrients.

All About Carbs 35

ALL OF THIS HYPE BEGS THE QUESTION—CAN WE EAT TOO FEW CARBS?

Entering ketosis comes at a price. Most of us require some level of carbs to function at our best. For example, lowering carbs makes us short of temper, affects our sleep, and limits our ability to train at high intensities.

Athletes vs. non-athletes

As we mentioned above, when it comes to calories, your body needs a certain amount of energy to function. For quick energy, carbs are the body's preferred source, as they produce the greatest amount of ATP (energy) per molecule. However, we don't always need maximum energy, such as when we're sitting on our couch watching TV.

The respiratory exchange ratio

A majority of our daily functions don't require a ton of energy. We're just sitting there, breathing normally, going about our business. As activity increases, so does our breathing rate. Our respiratory exchange ratio (RER), or the ratio between the amount of carbon dioxide produced by metabolism to the amount of oxygen used, determines what type of fuel we need. Under healthy metabolic conditions, RER fluctuates between 0.7 and 1.0.

At rest or during lower-intensity exercise, the body runs primarily on stored fats, showing a typical RER around 0.7. As exercise intensity and breathing rate increase, the body shifts toward carbohydrate use. RER values approaching 1.0 indicate carbs are being used as the primary fuel source. Research shows that training at or above 85 percent of maximum oxygen uptake meets these requirements.

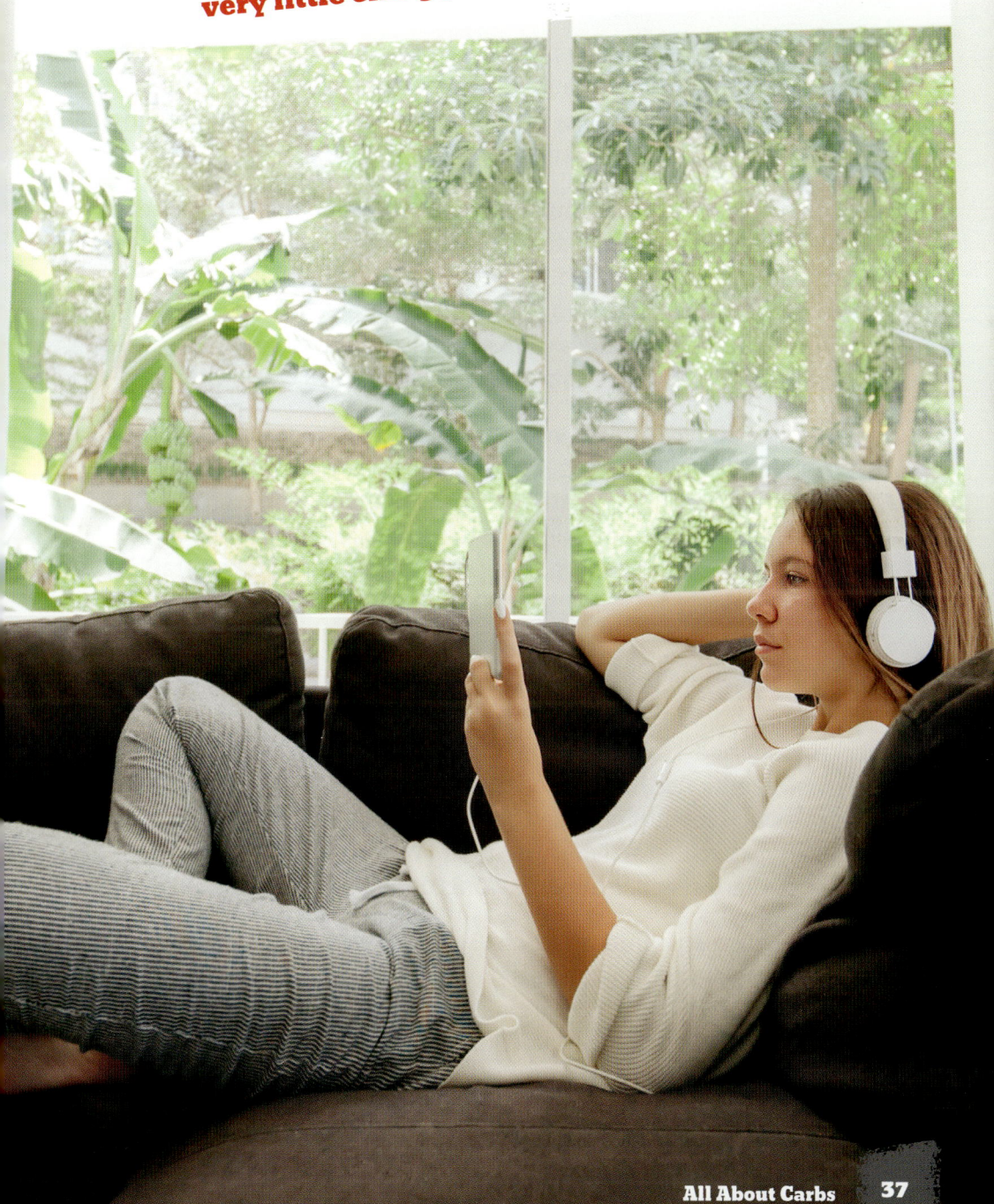

For most people, normal life requires very little energy.

Carbs for non-athletes

Why does all of this matter? In theory, one could fuel "regular life" on fats alone, assuming you never needed to exert yourself. Fats fuel low- to moderate-intensity exercise as well, such as slow distance running. So how does this affect your brain?

In the short term, low-carb diets have been shown to reduce memory and reaction time. That's because the human brain prefers glucose as its energy source. So, if you've got a big test coming up, or simply want to do well on your homework, eating carbs can help.

However, these effects are temporary. As the brain adapts to low-carb eating, it begins to produce ketones *en masse*. This shift was originally the goal of the Atkins diet—reducing the levels of glutamate in the brain to stop seizures. According to a study in the *Archives of Internal Medicine*, researchers found no difference in cognitive function between those who ate low- or high-carb diets in the long term.

However, the above results have been found in adults. For adolescents whose brains are still growing, carbs provide a key energy source. Furthermore, foods high in carbs are also full of micronutrients—folate, B vitamins, calcium, and iron, to name a few. To get enough of these vitamins and minerals, adolescents should eat fruit, vegetables, and whole grains.

Carbs for athletes

Any athlete who wants to fuel performance needs carbs. When we eat carbs, our bodies work hard to break carbs down into glucose. As previously mentioned, low-intensity exercise uses glucose and fats for energy through something called aerobic metabolism. Assuming there's enough oxygen to fuel activity, we can carry on producing energy in this manner. It's very effective but only works under low demand.

Therefore, as exercise intensity increases, such as during athletic events, we need energy faster. Thanks to a process known as **glycolysis**, the body can break down glucose without oxygen. You may have learned a little about it in your biology class. But in short, when intensity is high enough, usually around 85 percent of your maximum oxygen uptake,

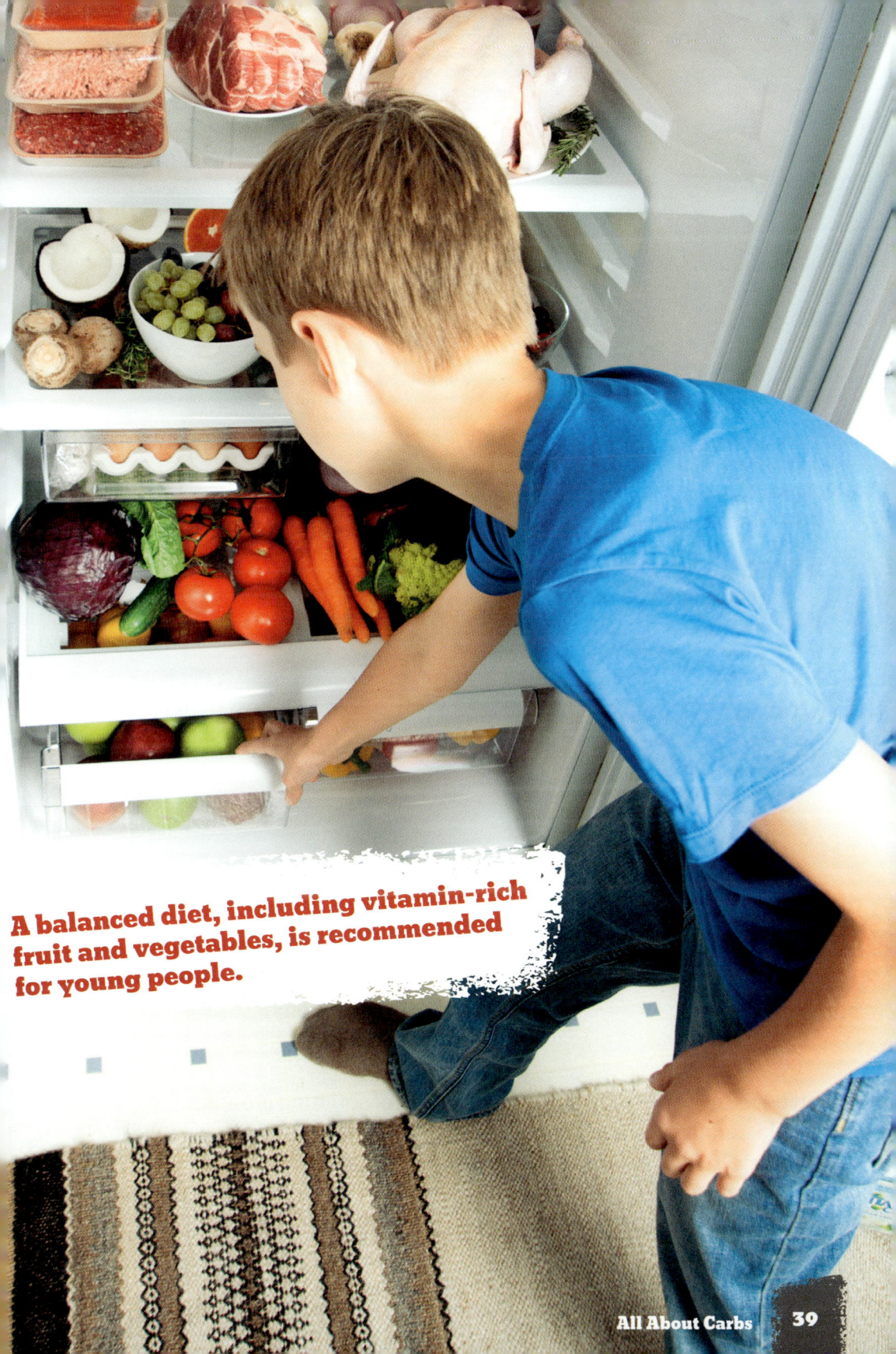

A balanced diet, including vitamin-rich fruit and vegetables, is recommended for young people.

All About Carbs 39

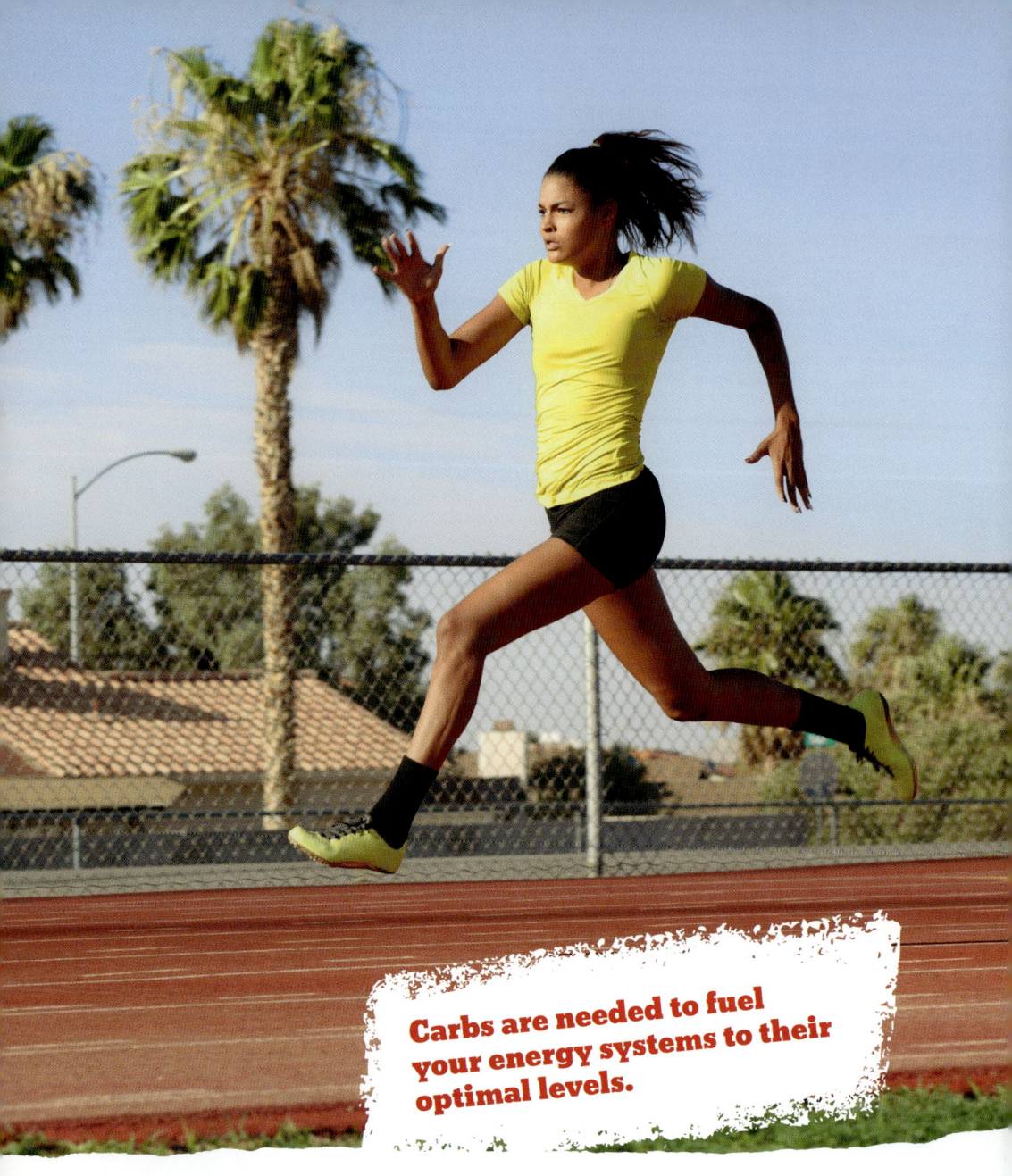

Carbs are needed to fuel your energy systems to their optimal levels.

you're completely reliant on carbs. Think of sprinting around a football field, running back to defend your goal, or winning a 400-m race. As any athlete is only as good as their weakest link, your ability to perform relies on the conditioning of all of your energy systems. And without carbs, you just can't get there.

Not only do carbs fuel athletic performance, but they also help preserve muscle. Sports break you down, literally. They require a breakdown of stored nutrients to fuel activity. If you haven't eaten properly around your training, there's a chance your body will reach into your muscle tissue. If athletes eat enough carbs throughout the day, it can draw upon glycogen stores, breaking it down into glucose. If that's not present, then your body can create it from proteins. As amino acids aren't readily stored for future energy use, your body pulls from the best source it has—muscle tissue.

Instead of further damaging muscle, athletes should eat a diet rich in carbs, especially around practices and games. Carbs provide necessary fuel for performance, recovery, and growth in athletes.

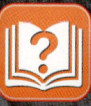

TEXT-DEPENDENT QUESTIONS

1. What is RER, and what does it have to do with your body's need for carbs?

2. Identify at least two reasons both athletes and non-athletes might need a diet rich in carbs.

3. What are the types of carbs, and how do they relate to their glycemic index?

RESEARCH PROJECT

Investigate the glycemic index of four or five of your favorite carbs. How would eating them right now affect your blood sugar? Based on what you read in the text, when would be the best time to add them to your meal? Put together a short paragraph on each.

WORDS TO UNDERSTAND

amino acids—the building blocks of proteins, made up of an amino group, a carboxyl group, a central carbon, and a side chain

anabolic—metabolic processes that build larger molecules, such as fats or body tissue, from smaller ones

autophagy—digestion of cellular constituents by enzymes of the same cell

branched-chain amino acids—amino acids with one central carbon chain bound to three or more carbons, whose chemical structure triggers important downstream processes, such as muscle protein synthesis

gluconeogenesis—the re-creation of glucose from non-carbohydrate carbon molecules, such as amino acids

mTOR pathway—a nutrient-sensing pathway that causes a domino effect in things like muscle growth, maturation, and metabolism

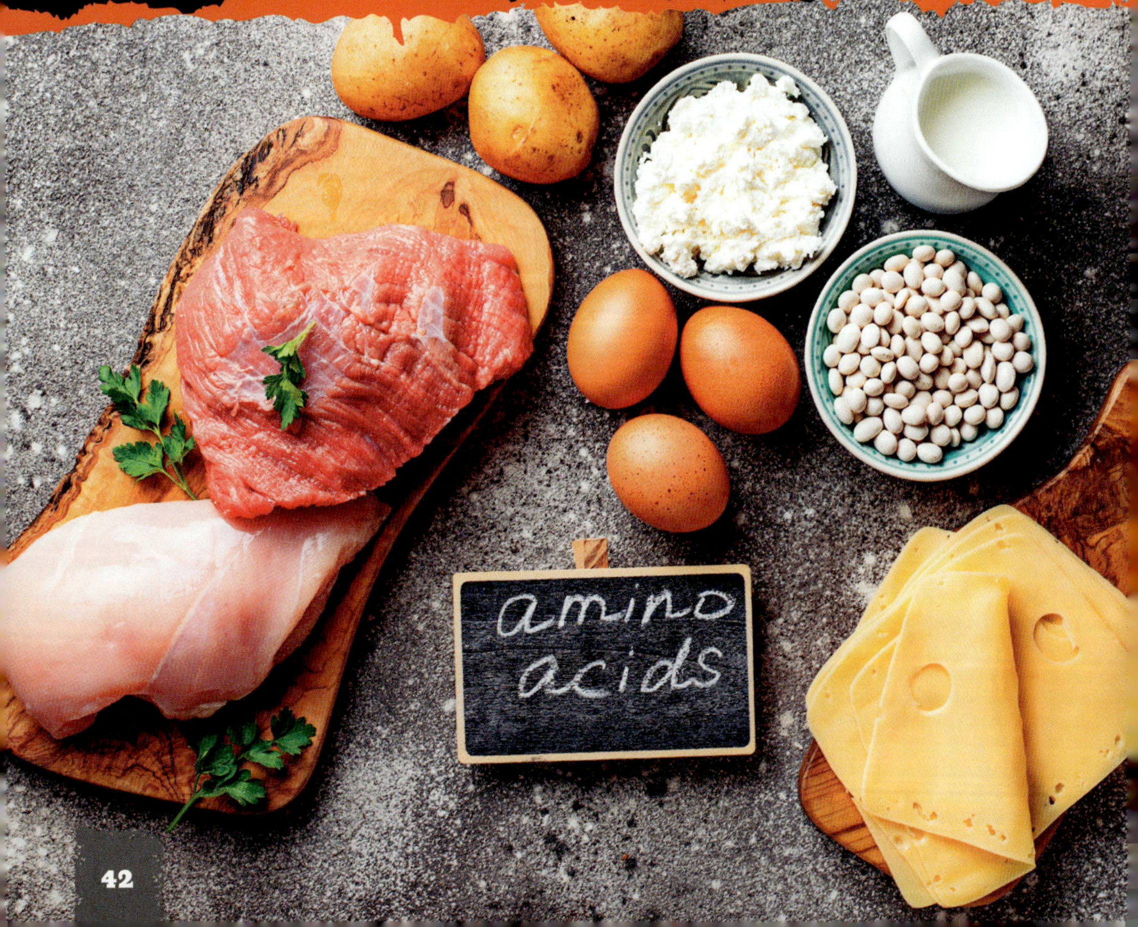

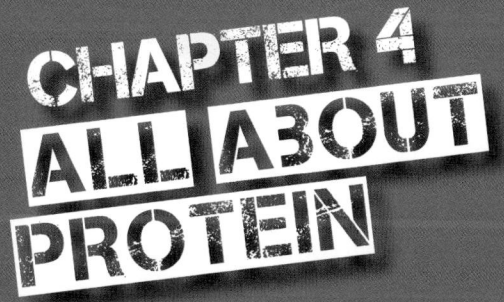

CHAPTER 4
ALL ABOUT PROTEIN

Protein is one of the four essential macronutrients (alongside water, fat, and carbs). It provides four calories of energy per gram, and it's become a hot topic in the health and fitness world. All of the most popular diets—low fat, Atkins, Keto, and Paleo—focus on high protein content. But what's so important about protein, and is it better for you than carbs or fats?

WHAT IS PROTEIN?

Structurally, proteins are made up of something called **amino acids**. Amino acids are compounds made up of an amino group, a carboxyl group, a central carbon, and a side chain. Without getting too deep into biochemistry, this means different proteins (with different amino acid structures) can serve different purposes. When you put all of these tiny building blocks together, you can create tissues like bone and muscle, enzymes that jump-start metabolism, hormones, and more. Therefore, without all of the necessary amino acids, your physiological functioning is limited.

We know we need protein—but how do you know how much is enough?

According to *Harvard Health*, the recommended daily allowance of protein is around 0.8 g/kg of body weight. However, depending on your activity level, other macronutrient intake, and growth rate, you could need up to 1.2–2 g/kg of body weight. Those with naturally more muscle mass, such as a college football player, will likely require more protein than an average twelve-year-old. Other factors such as injury status, activity level, and age play a role in protein requirements. Higher protein intake is linked to better metabolism, higher sports performance, and healthy weight management.

Non-essential vs. essential amino acids

The human body contains 20 amino acids that build the proteins that support your daily life. Not all of them, however, are considered essential. Essential amino acids are those you have to obtain from your diet. Nine out of the twenty need to come from food, while your body can make the rest.

Eating certain amino acids can even trigger **anabolic** processes, such as muscle protein synthesis. For example, the three **branched-chain amino acids** (BCAAs)—leucine, isoleucine, and valine—can accelerate

Amino acids are used in the body to build proteins.

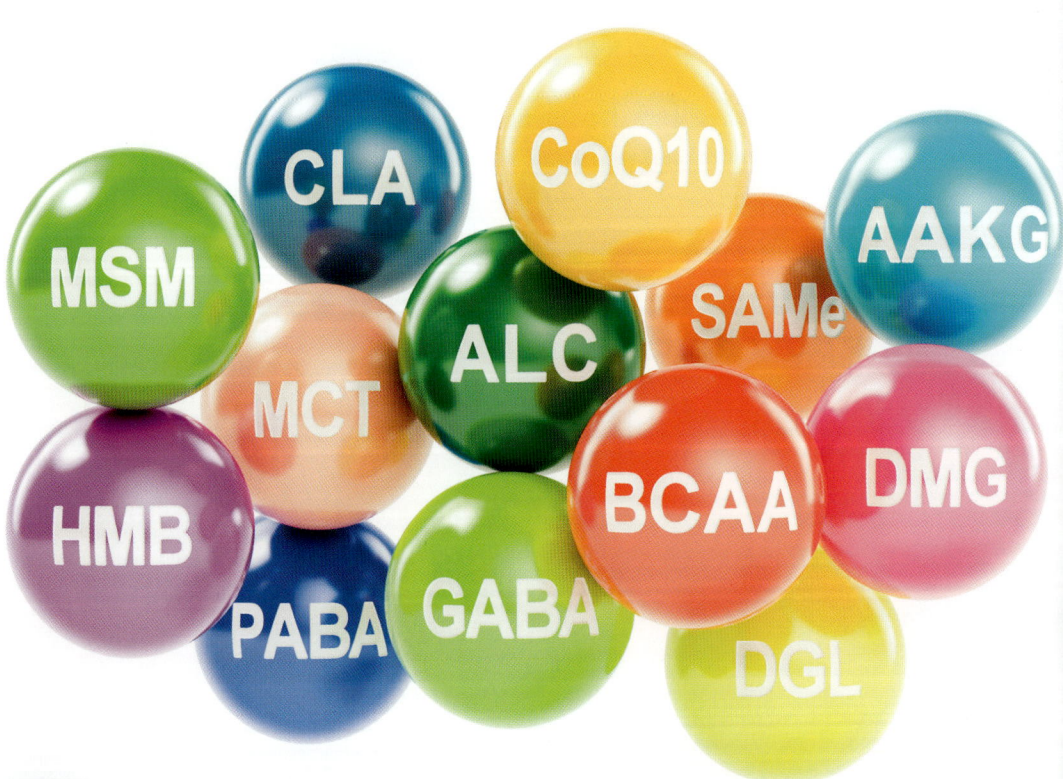

Fitness and Nutrition

muscle growth after exercise. That doesn't mean taking them will make you a bodybuilder, but they can definitely help you recover and prevent soreness.

The following is a list of essential amino acids, including their uses and dietary sources:

- Histidine
    - Precursor to histamine
    - Plays a role in the growth and function of immune cells
    - Absence of histidine/histamine can result in chronic fatigue and infection
    - Dietary sources: beans, meat, seafood, dairy products, brown rice, poultry, and rye
- Isoleucine
    - Increases muscular uptake of glucose for glycogen stores, which is important to muscle growth
    - Signals the onset of muscle protein synthesis (with leucine)
    - Dietary sources: dairy products, fish, almonds, chicken, cashews, and soy
- Leucine
    - Identified as the most important BCAA for muscle protein synthesis, especially through the **mTOR pathway**
    - Regulates protein turnover by preventing protein breakdown
    - Increases insulin response
    - Acts as a shuttle for ammonia in **gluconeogenesis**
    - Crucial to energy regulation and wound healing
    - Dietary sources: cheese, chicken, lamb, steak, tuna, and pumpkin
- Lysine
    - Required for growth and tissue repair
    - Breakdown of lysine forms acetyl-CoA, which facilitates carbohydrate metabolism

- - Generates connective tissue and bone
  - Dietary sources: lentils, tofu, legumes, and quinoa
- Methionine
  - A precursor to creatine—levels of methionine set upper limit on creatine phosphate, the primary fuel for short, intense exercise
  - Dietary sources: egg, brazil nuts, beef, cheese, chicken, and turkey
- Phenylalanine
  - Highly prevalent in the brain
  - Synthesizes tyrosine to produce neurotransmitters
  - Dietary sources: pork, chicken, yogurt, and turkey
- Threonine
  - Produces glycine and serine, which are important for cell growth; basically you need to eat enough threonine so the body can produce these other amino acids on its own
  - Contributes to muscle tissue generation
  - Crucial to immune system function
  - Dietary sources: eggs, gelatin, milk, fish, bananas, and carrots
- Tryptophan
  - Enables production of cellular energy
  - Synthesizes NAD+ and NADP, which are critical to metabolism and energy production
  - Dietary sources: flaxseed, salami, turkey, chicken, and eggs
- Valine
  - Anabolic in the stimulation of muscle tissue synthesis
  - Contributes to glucose uptake in muscle by activating insulin
  - Prevents tissue breakdown
  - Dietary sources: milk, beef, chicken, and chickpeas

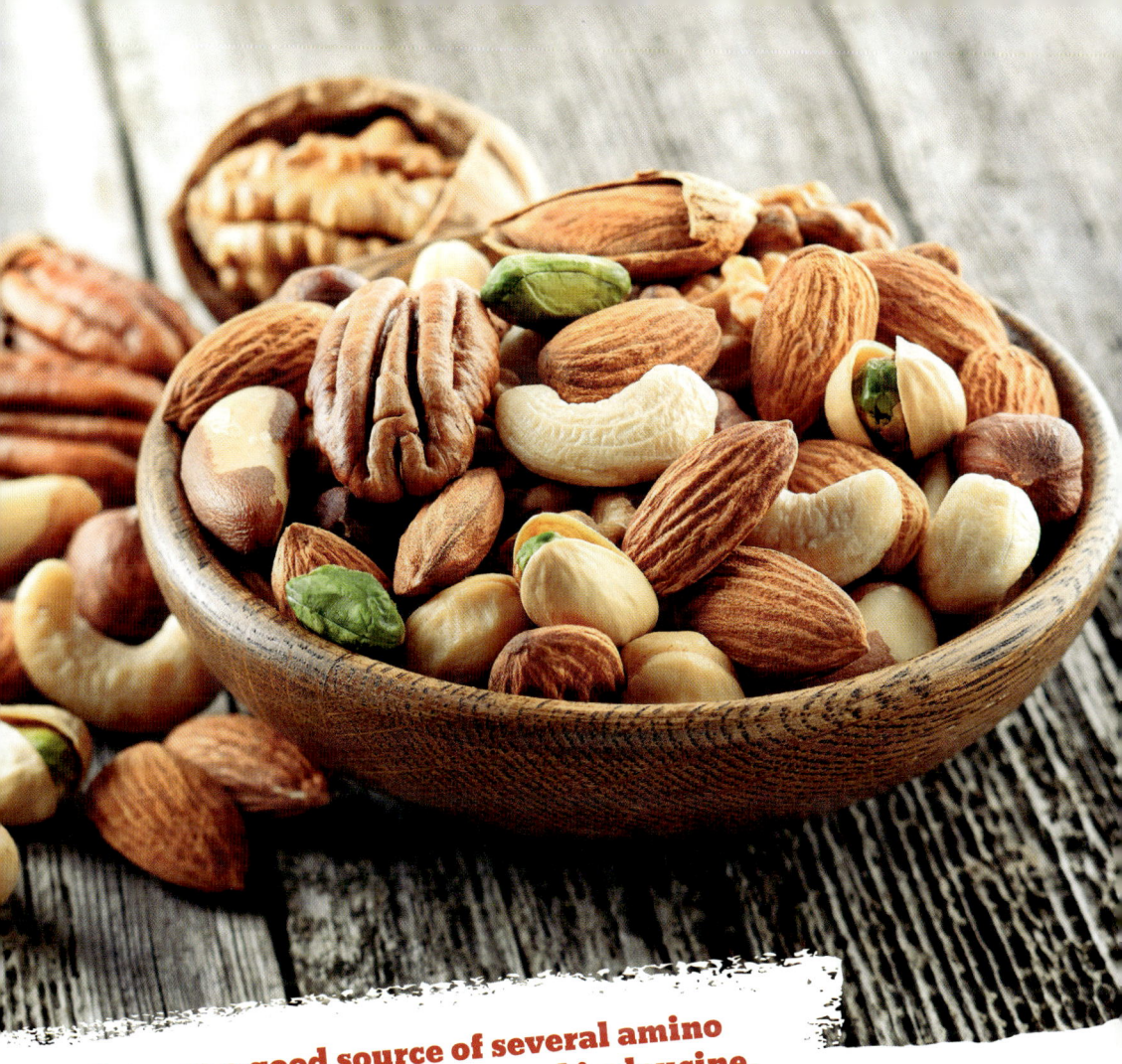

Nuts are a good source of several amino acids, such as methionine and isoleucine.

Despite their name, non-essential amino acids still serve a purpose. The term simply means that the human body can synthesize them by itself. For example, alanine is made from a byproduct of glucose metabolism (pyruvate), and the precursor to tyrosine is another amino acid—phenylalanine. Just because we can make them doesn't mean they don't have value in our diet. Under extreme conditions, some non-essential amino acids can become essential, especially if we're lacking in nutrients elsewhere.

Below is a list of non-essential amino acids, their purpose, and common dietary sources:

- Alanine
  - Important for amino acid metabolism
  - Made from lactic acid, so it balances pH
  - Can be used to produce glucose in the absence of carbs
  - Dietary sources: seafood, beef, beans, nuts, and eggs
- Arginine
  - Conditionally essential during illness or severe stress
  - Supports immune function and circulation
  - Activates mTOR pathway for protein synthesis
  - Dietary sources: turkey, chicken, pork, peanuts, soybeans, walnuts, almonds, tuna, lentils, and salmon
- Asparagine
  - A precursor to aspartic acid
  - Dietary sources (see *aspartic acid*)
- Aspartic acid
  - Builds intermediates for cellular metabolism
  - Can assist in aerobic recovery
  - Dietary sources: dairy, whey protein, beef, legumes, nuts, and seafood
- Cysteine
  - Reduces inflammation from exercise
  - A precursor to thyroid hormone T4, which helps with metabolic activity, protein synthesis, and growth
  - Dietary sources: poultry, cheese, fish, brazil nuts, soybeans, and oats

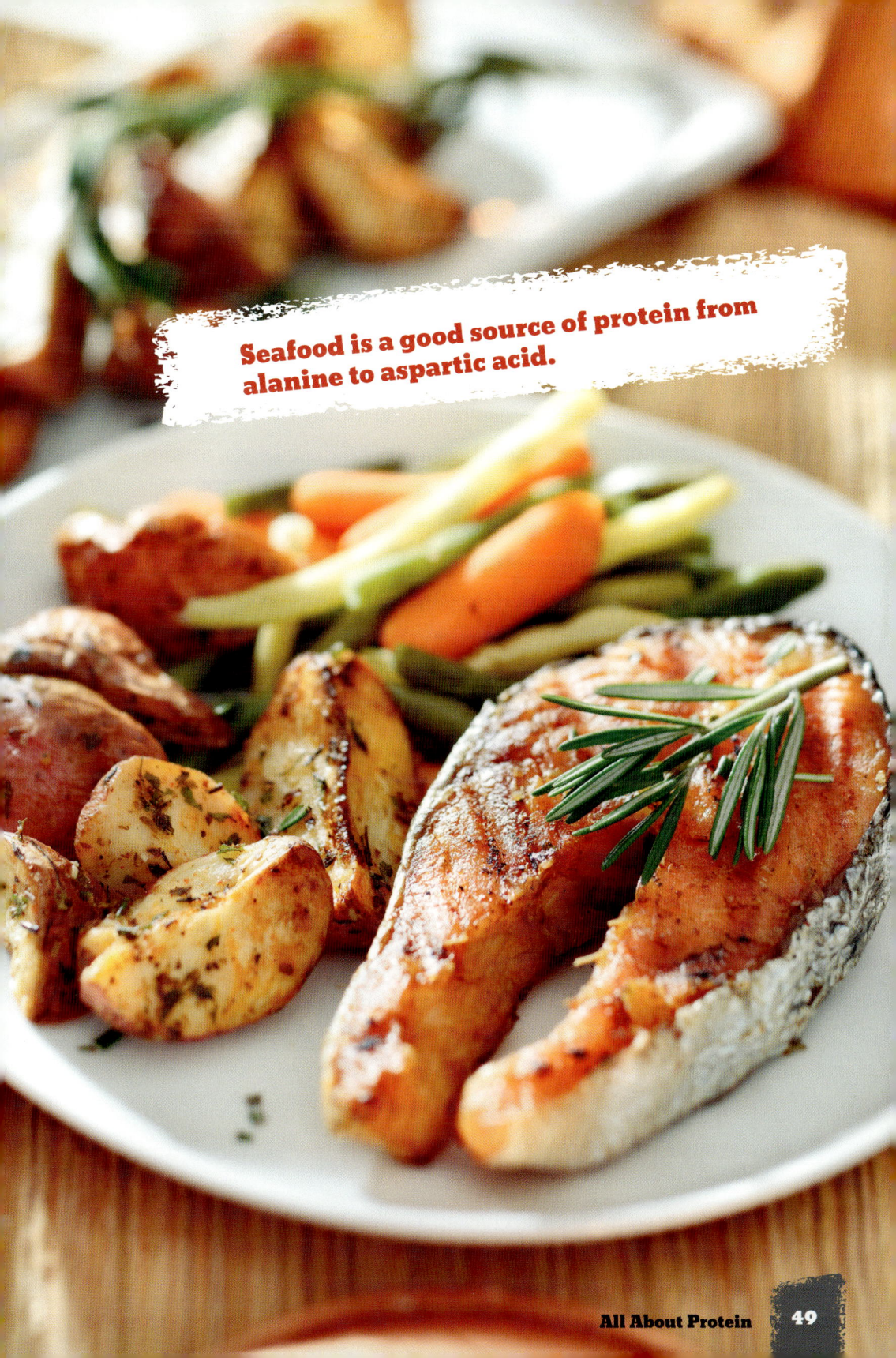

Seafood is a good source of protein from alanine to aspartic acid.

- Glutamic acid
    - Promotes muscle growth during caloric restriction through assisting gluconeogenesis
    - Manufactures glutamine
    - Dietary sources: soy protein, seeds, eggs, cod fish, and cheese
- Glutamine
    - Conditionally essential in cases of heavy training
    - Synthesizes peptides and tissue healing
    - Can help remove waste and nitrogen from muscle tissue
    - Dietary sources: chicken, beef, dairy products, eggs, certain vegetables such as spinach, carrots, and brussel sprouts
- Glycine
    - Aids in the synthesis of collagen
    - Dietary sources: fish, dairy, meat, beans, pumpkin, and cauliflower
- Proline
    - Forms amino acids that make up connective tissue such as tendons and ligaments
    - Dietary sources: gelatin, cottage cheese, and beef
- Serine
    - Helps in the formation of blood vessels
    - Prevalent in cell membranes as it builds proteins and enzymes that control cellular transfer
    - Dietary sources: meat, fish, barley, and white beans; serine can be derived from protein and phospholipid degradation as well as dietary sources
- Tyrosine
    - A precursor to dopamine, norepinephrine, and epinephrine
    - Through building catecholamines, raises senses, mood, and overall readiness
    - Dietary sources: pork, chicken, yogurt, and turkey

 The importance of protein is examined in this short video.

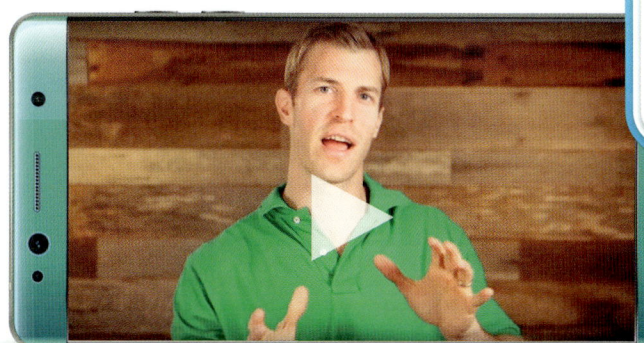

Tyrosine is used in the body to build chemicals that regulate mood and movement.

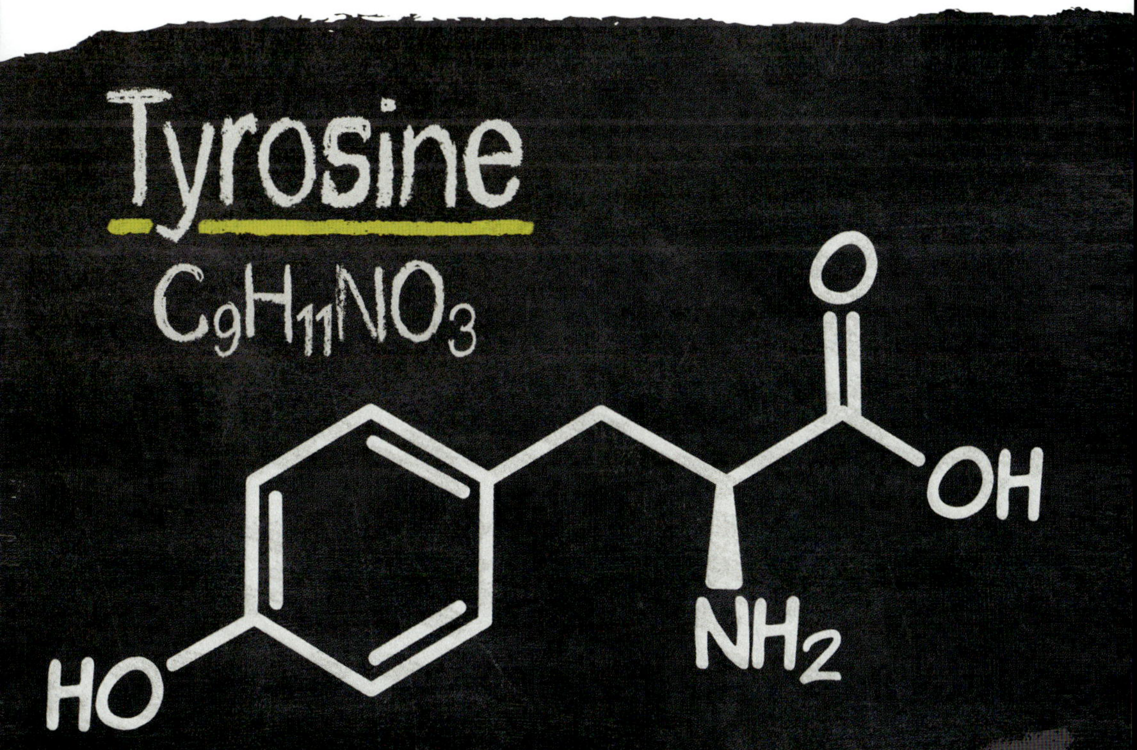

Tyrosine
$C_9H_{11}NO_3$

BENEFITS OF DIETARY PROTEIN

As you can see from this extensive list, the human body relies on amino acids, and therefore protein, for a *ton* of metabolic activity. That's why all balanced diets focus on adequate protein intake first. By eating protein, you can expect a healthy metabolism, along with muscle growth, appetite control, and accelerated healing.

Increased muscle mass

BCAAs enhance the rate of muscle protein synthesis. On top of resistance exercise, ingesting post-workout protein compounds the anabolic effect. Leucine, in particular, activates the mTOR pathway, a cell signaling process that regulates cell growth, increase, survival, protein synthesis, **autophagy**, and transcription. According to research, 20 g of post-exercise leucine-dominant BCAA supplementation maximizes muscle growth after resistance training.

Reduced appetite

Protein has been shown to slow how quickly the stomach empties, making you feel full longer. Unlike high-glycemic carbs, it won't rapidly

PROTEIN IN PLANT-BASED DIETS

Diets in which protein tends to be a concern are the vegetarian or vegan diet. Plant-based foods have huge nutritional benefits for their fiber, vitamins, minerals, and more. Yet fruit and vegetables are low in protein. So, can you get enough protein on a plant-based diet? As it turns out—yes, you can. As long as you diversify your meals, it's completely possible to get a balanced amino acid profile. Tofu, brown rice, beans, legumes, wheat, oats, nuts, and even peas are all rich in amino acids. Try combining these on your plate, and work with a nutritionist if you have any concerns.

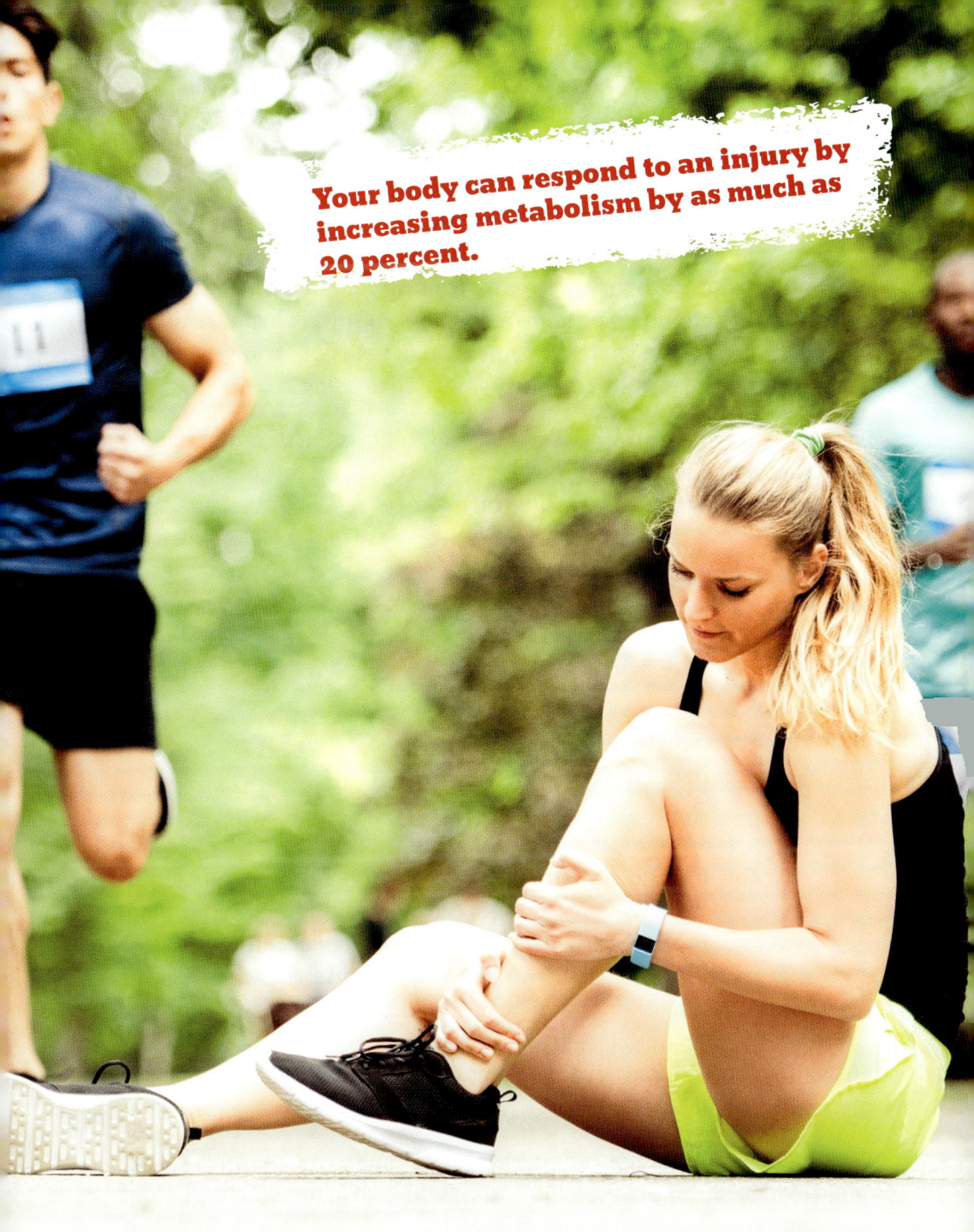

Your body can respond to an injury by increasing metabolism by as much as 20 percent.

raise your blood sugar or decrease insulin sensitivity. Therefore, you safely can add protein powder to your snacks or meals while limiting the total caloric intake and hormonal response.

Injury repair

Whether it's a sports injury or simply scraping your knee, overcoming injury requires adequate protein. Your metabolism can increase up to 20 percent due to injury. Therefore, you need to eat enough to match this healing response, despite training volume decreasing.

Fortunately, if you're an athlete who already follows the recommended protein intake (1.2–2 g/kg body weight), you should be covered. However, specific supplemental amino acids can make cell repair faster. Glutamine and arginine are conditionally essential at times of injury. Make sure to get more foods with these two when recovering, such as chicken, eggs, walnuts, almonds, salmon, and dairy.

IF PROTEIN IS SO GOOD FOR US, CAN WE EAT TOO MUCH?

Yes, you can have too much protein. Although many diets such as Keto and Paleo advocate for high protein intake, your total caloric intake includes all macronutrients. If you stick to the same daily caloric intake, overeating protein takes away from carbs/fats. Not getting adequate amounts of fats and carbs in your diet can actually slow your progress. Fats are critical for recovery, as they make up the lining of your cells and provide lasting fuel. Carbs are stored in muscle and are the body's preferred source of energy. So, without enough carbs, your body is going to go searching in other places, potentially breaking down muscle in the process.

On the other hand, simply adding more protein *to* your current intake could lead to chronic overeating and weight gain in underactive people. So, what do you do? Shoot for between 1.2–2 g/kg of body weight, and adjust your fat and carb content according to your exercise schedule. More aerobic and high-intensity lifting warrants more carbs; rest and light days warrant more fats; and resistance training should always be supplemented with protein.

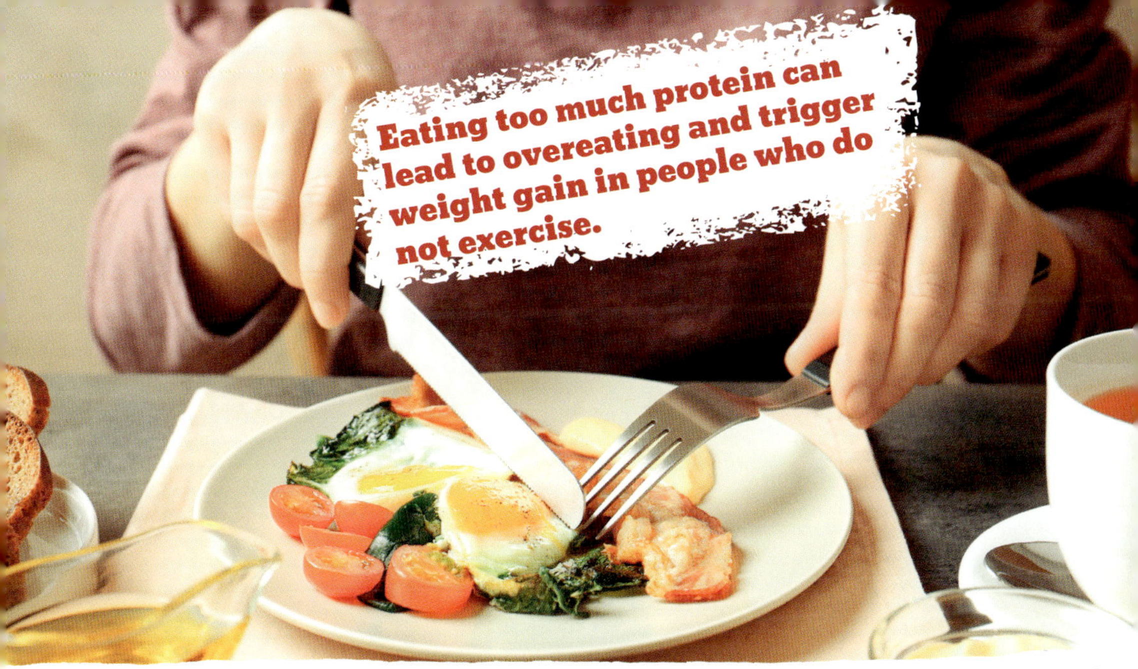

> Eating too much protein can lead to overeating and trigger weight gain in people who do not exercise.

TEXT-DEPENDENT QUESTIONS

1. Name at least three amino acids involved in injury repair, and include the foods from which you can get them.

2. What factors play a role in your daily protein requirements, and how can you make sure you're getting enough?

3. What are the benefits of adding protein to your meals, alongside other macronutrients?

RESEARCH PROJECT

The nutritional value of any dietary protein can be scored against something called the PDCAAS—protein digestibility-corrected amino acid scores. Research, compare, and contrast the PDCAAS of 4–5 proteins, including at least one vegetarian source. How might this score affect your meal choice depending on your lifestyle? Put together a short argument featuring a table or graphic to defend your answer.

WORDS TO UNDERSTAND

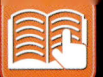

adipose tissue—also known as body fat, it's a tissue naturally found all around the human body necessary for cushioning, energy storage, and insulation

monounsaturated fats—fats with one double bond at the end of their fatty acid chain

polyunsaturated fats—fats whose hydrocarbon chains contain multiple double bonds in their chemical structure, and are typically liquid at room temperature

saturated fats—a type of fat with a long hydrocarbon chain whose bonds are saturated with hydrogen, and are typically solid at room temperature

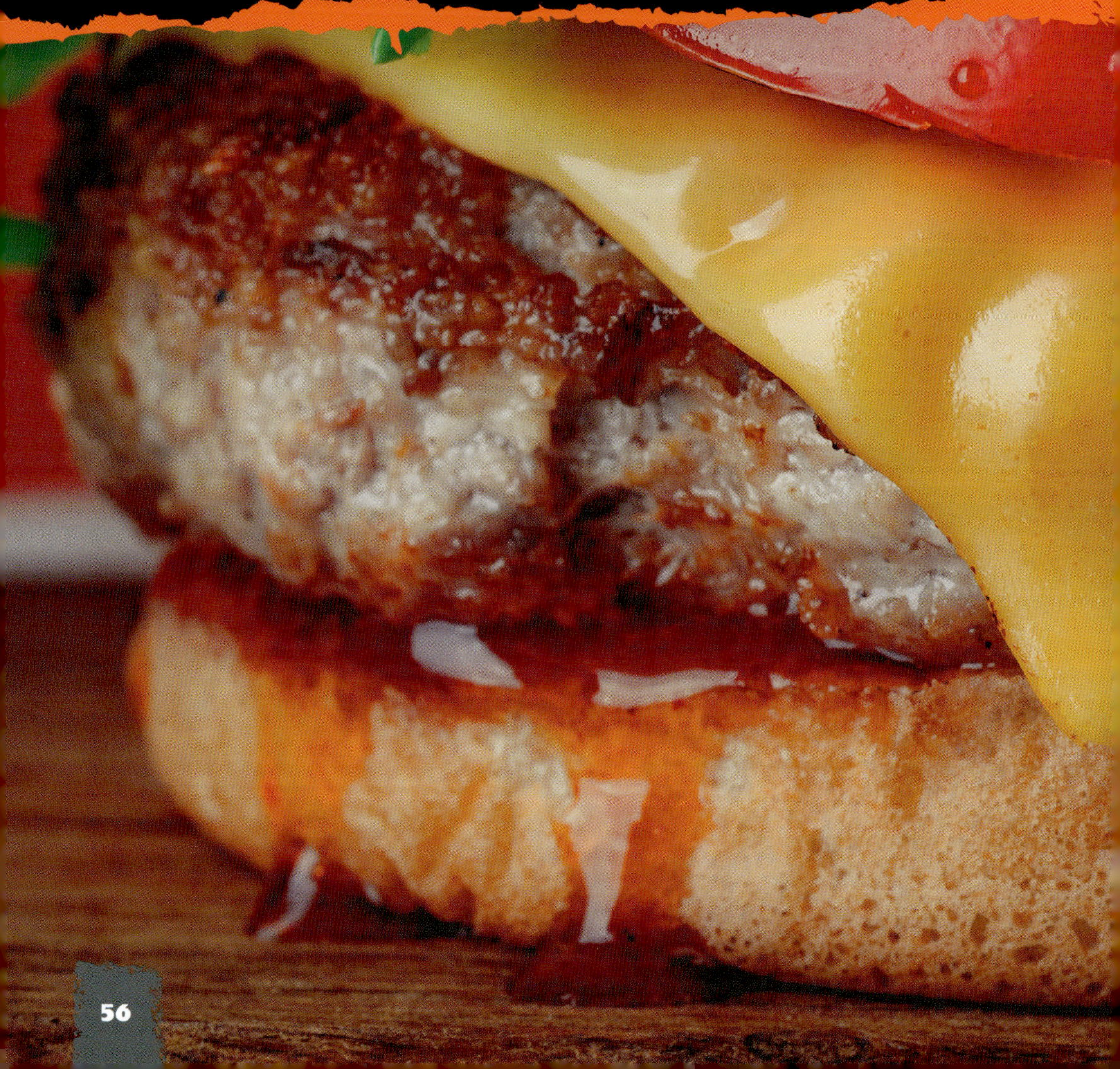

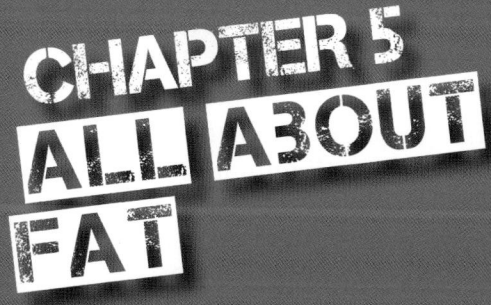

CHAPTER 5
ALL ABOUT FAT

WHAT IS FAT?

When you think of fat, what comes to mind?

For many, it's the extra weight humans carry on their bodies as a result of bad diet and/or lack of exercise, and is something to avoid. This thinking is largely flawed. In fact, fats are a vital part of a healthy diet!

The tissue commonly known as body fat is actually **adipose tissue**. Adipose tissue is naturally found all around the human body, from underneath the skin to surrounding your organs. It's even in bone marrow! Some amount of adipose tissue is a requirement for health, despite the shadow often cast upon it by the fitness industry. It insulates the body against the elements, cushions organs from crashing into each other, and stores energy for later use.

To make a long story short—we need body fat! Dietary fats can contribute to a healthy level of body fat. Simply eating food rich in fat doesn't necessarily add to your adipose tissue. Eating fat doesn't make you fat—it's much more complicated than that.

DIFFERENT TYPES OF DIETARY FATS

There are four different types of dietary fats—monounsaturated, polyunsaturated, saturated, and trans fats. These variations are due to their distinct chemical structure. **Monounsaturated fats** have one double bond at the end of their fatty acid chain (hence the term "mono"). **Polyunsaturated fats** have multiple double bonds, while **saturated fats** have no double bonds since they're saturated with hydrogen atoms.

Similar to carbs, these differences in their chemical structure yield different interactions within the human body. The "right" kinds of fats can make cells more fluid, able to change quickly, and adaptable. The "wrong" kinds lead to heart disease, obesity, inflammation, and more.

WHICH FATS ARE CONSIDERED "GOOD FATS"?

The good fats are monounsaturated and polyunsaturated. Monounsaturated fats are typically common in healthy diets such as the Mediterranean diet, which is low in saturated fats. Polyunsaturated fats are even more essential. Our bodies need them to build cell membranes, cover neurons, and stop bleeding. However, we can't make them on our own. Therefore, we rely on our diet to provide vital lipids for cellular health, brain function, and chemical messengers.

Good fats build strong cell membranes

The cells within the human body are encased by a lipid bilayer. This membrane is composed of two layers of fats stacked atop each other, forming a semipermeable, polar barrier. This structure allows for selective protection of the cell, maintaining its shape, letting the right nutrients in, and keeping the wrong stuff out.

Good fats help our brains function properly

The brain is composed primarily of fats, whose structures are composed of omega-3 fatty acids. According to one comprehensive 2016 study, an omega-3 fatty acid found especially in fish of cold waters, as well as in the human brain, called docosahexaenoic acid (DHA) by itself, contributes to "modulating signal transduction pathways, neurotransmission, neurogenesis, myelination, membrane receptor function, synaptic plasticity, neuroinflammation, membrane integrity

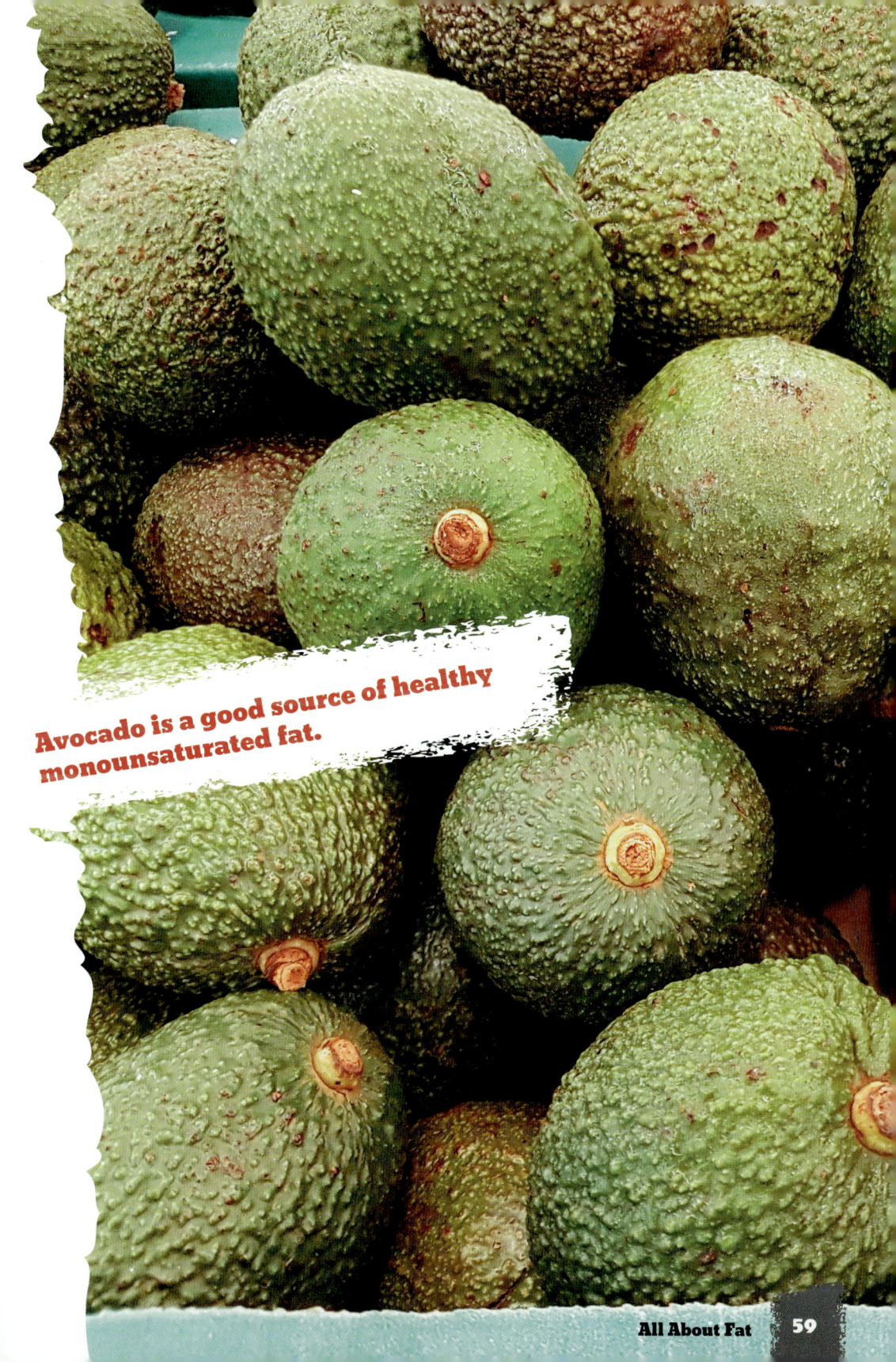

Avocado is a good source of healthy monounsaturated fat.

and membrane organization." In layman's terms, that means that a little fat can help you think clearer and faster, generate new brain cells, learn new function and habits, quell inflammation, and keep the integrity of your neurons.

Good fats help counteract inflammation

Exercise, psychological pressure, and other stressors can cause elevations in cortisol, the stress hormone. In the short term, this narrows our attention span and accelerates our metabolism so we can react appropriately. Cortisol helps us run faster, focus more, and think sharper. It also triggers inflammation to start the healing

Elevated levels of cortisol in the body can lead to chronic inflammation.

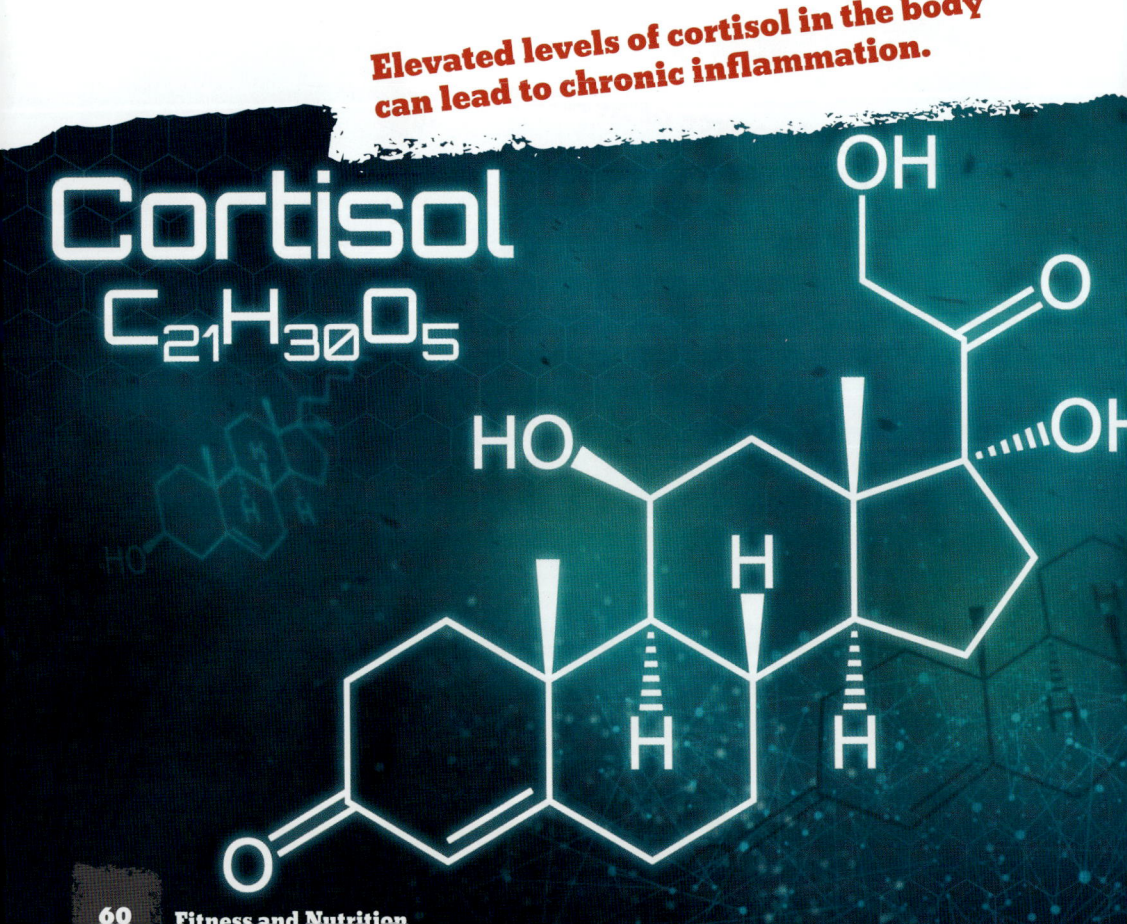

Cortisol $C_{21}H_{30}O_5$

process from those high demands. However, chronic stress leads to continued elevation of cortisol, and therefore chronic inflammation. Omega-3 fats help block the pathways in the body that cause inflammation, therefore decreasing it. Much like you'd apply rest, ice, elevation, and compression for an acute joint injury, these fats can be applied for chronic inflammation.

WHICH FATS ARE CONSIDERED "BAD FATS"?

On the other side of the coin lie saturated fats and trans fats. Commonly referred to as "bad" fats, these types can negatively impact your health when consumed in large quantities.

Saturated fats

An imbalanced diet of saturated fats to unsaturated fats is associated with cardiovascular disease. According to the *American Journal of Clinical Nutrition*, the replacement of saturated fats with mono- and polyunsaturated fats reduces high cholesterol levels. However, simply removing saturated fats isn't enough—when replaced with refined carbs, the risk of developing clogged arteries and high cholesterol remained. Recent research even shows that certain types of saturated fats, such as medium-chain triglycerides, are associated with better metabolism, exercise endurance, and decreased body fat.

Evidence exists that humans have safely consumed a balance of poly-, mono-, and saturated fats throughout history. It's only thanks to modern Western lifestyles that diets have shifted toward saturated fats, and unnatural ones at that. Instead, you should aim for an equal distribution.

Due to a strong level of research on the risks of saturated fats, however, the American Heart Association strongly recommends an intake of no more than 5–6 percent of total daily calories. Foods containing saturated fats include whole-fat dairy, beef, coconut oil, and pork.

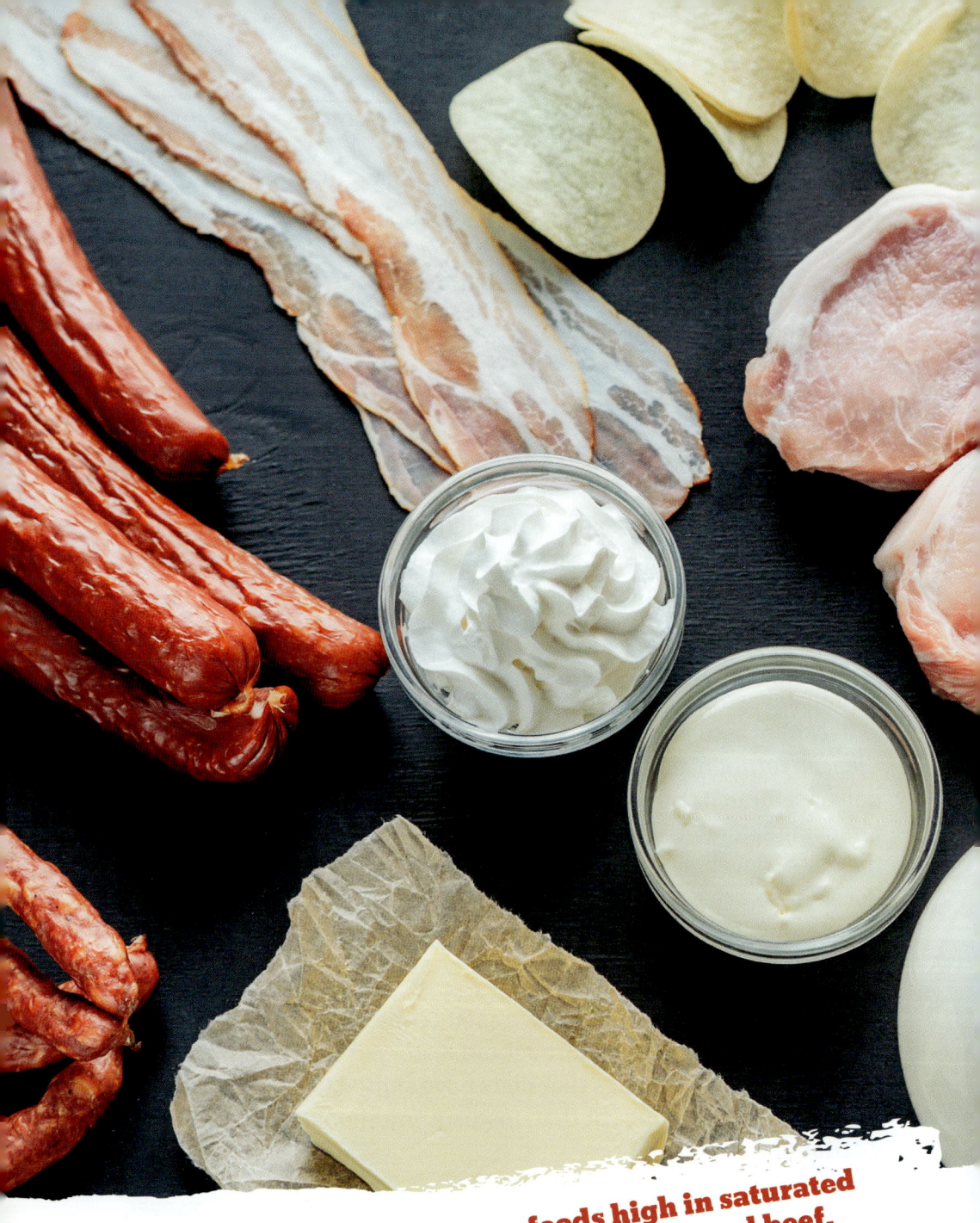

A diet of too many foods high in saturated fats, such as whole milk, pork, and beef, can lead to cholesterol problems.

While saturated fats aren't ALL evil, there is one type of fat that is—trans-fat.

Trans fats

Trans fats were made by humans to prolong shelf life. If you looked at the nutrition facts of processed foods, you might see trans fats denoted as "partially hydrogenated vegetable oils." Basically manufacturers create them by adding excess hydrogen atoms to the structure of vegetable oils. This process is called **hydrogenation**.

Normally fatty acids are composed of long chains of hydrocarbons that can fold upon themselves. Trans fats, on the other hand, do not fold. Therefore, they can pack really tightly into cell membranes, essentially destroying their fluidity and function.

According to the *British Medical Journal*, a high intake of trans fats increases the risk of death from coronary heart disease by 28 percent, and the risk of ANY death by 34 percent. It's suggested that trans fats do so by raising blood levels of lipoproteins and triglycerides—two compounds that clog arteries. Finally, trans fats can even compete with essential fats, the ones you need to build healthy cell membranes and improve brain function. Trans fat intake has a high correlation with heart disease as it destroys the elasticity of cells. Fried foods and others

CAN CARBS BE CONVERTED TO FAT?

Consuming too many carbs without adequate exercise levels can lead to increased body fat. With nowhere to go, the excess blood glucose found in carbs is converted to triglycerides, a type of fat found within the body, and stored as adipose tissue. As fats contain more calories per gram, they allow for more efficient energy storage—sort of like renting out a bigger storage unit instead of trying to cram all of your stuff in. Plus, fats are ideal to fuel resting metabolic activity. And, in the absence of an active lifestyle, that's most of the fuel you need.

 **Find out why all fat is not created equal.**

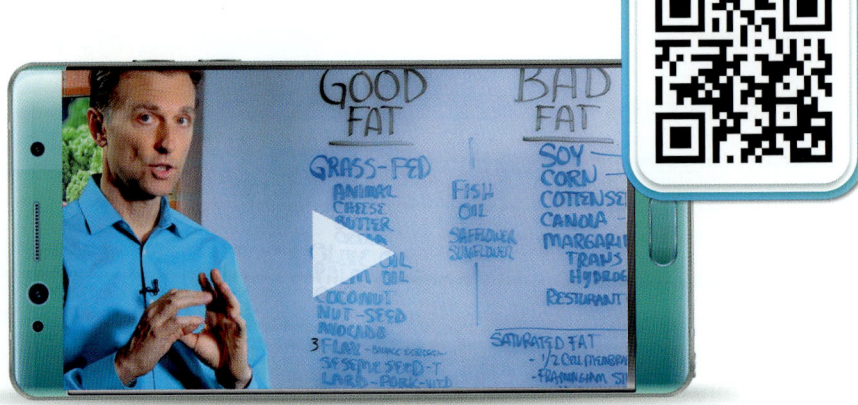

containing hydrogenated oils can cause blood vessel inflammation, so avoid them if possible.

DO WE GET FAT BY EATING FAT?

Fats have a lot of calories per gram. When we eat too much of them, we run the risk of going over total caloric intake. Chronic overconsumption of calories, regardless of their source, can lead to fat gain. Eating too much trans fats can clog your arteries and destroy cell function, slowing your metabolism in the process. A slow metabolism combined with overindulgence and little exercise means our bodies are left with excess energy. In that case, it assumes we're saving up for some later emergency when food will be scarce. As such, it will store that extra energy as fat.

However, simply eating fat does not make you fat. As you've read in this chapter, good fats are critical for biological processes. In fact, their high caloric content can make us feel full *before* we overeat. Sugars, on the other hand, cause a quick energy spike without really filling us up. When that energy isn't used immediately for exercise

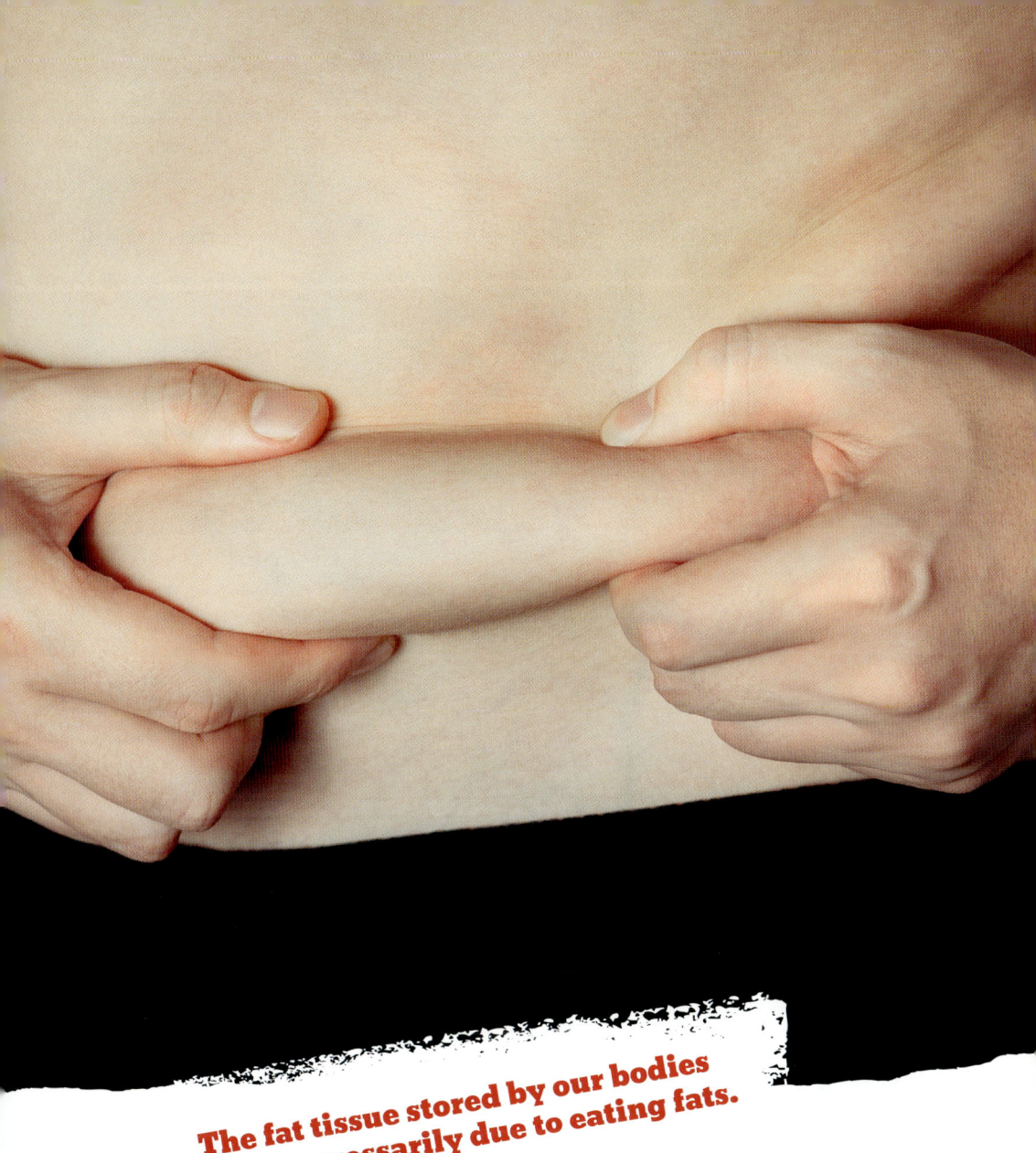

The fat tissue stored by our bodies is not necessarily due to eating fats.

or saved as glycogen, it's stored as fat. Even eating too much protein can lead to fat storage. It all comes down to overeating. As long as you control your caloric intake and view food as fuel, you don't have to worry.

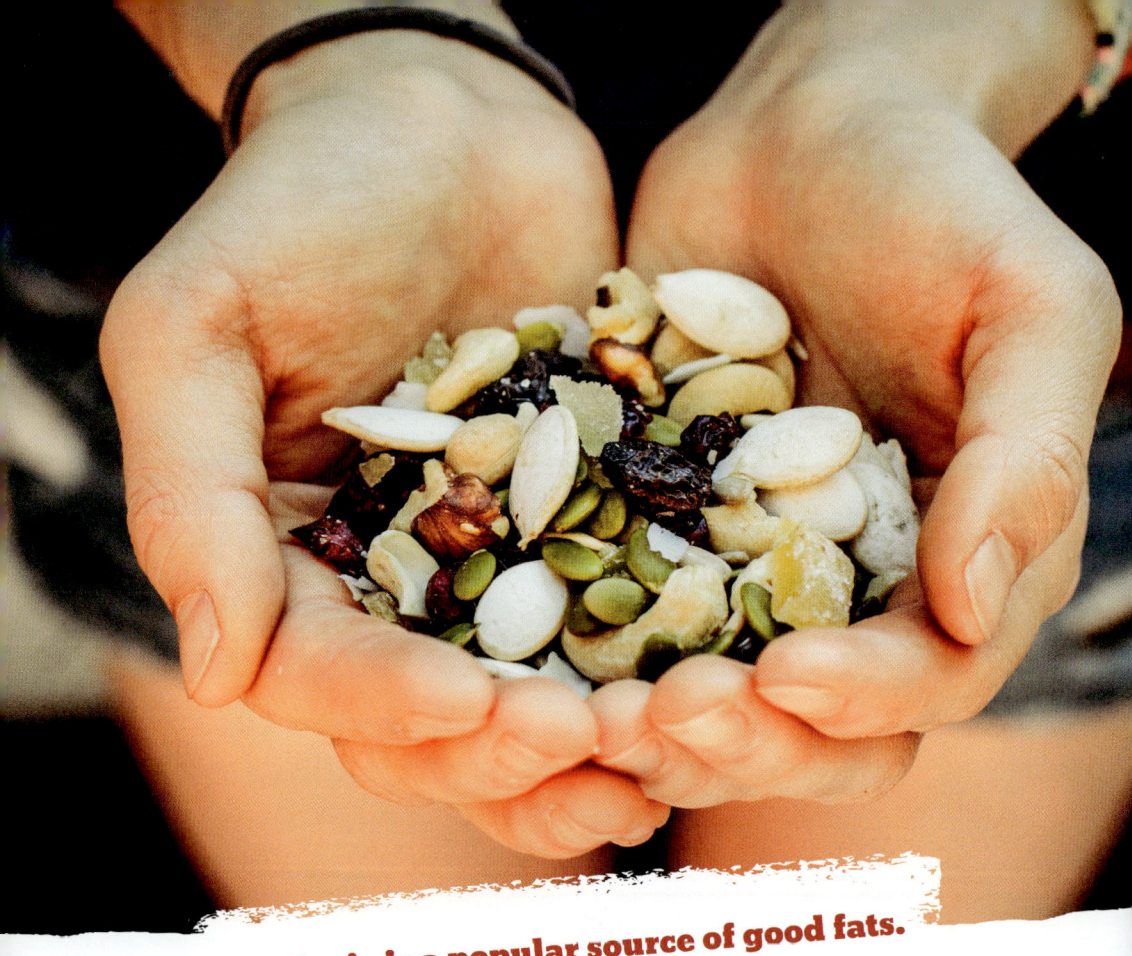

Trail mix is a popular source of good fats.

RECOMMENDATIONS FOR DAILY FAT INTAKE

Every person is different, but as a general guideline, remember to get at least one serving of at least three of these good fat sources every day:

- Mixed nut/trail mix
- 1 tablespoon of olive oil
- 6 ounces of fish and/or 2 g of fish oils
- Half an avocado (or a serving of guacamole)
- 6 ounces of flax seeds and/or 1 tablespoon of flaxseed oil

 Not all fat is bad for you. Watch this to learn what and how much to eat.

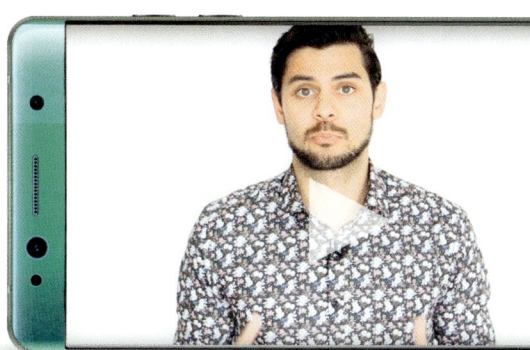

TEXT-DEPENDENT QUESTIONS

1. Which types of foods contain good fats, and what are the benefits of eating them?

2. What are trans fats and the risks associated with them?

3. Can eating fat make us fat? Be sure to include other factors that come into play to answer that question.

RESEARCH PROJECT

Pick two common meals (spaghetti and meatballs, burgers and fries, rice and beans, pizza, etc.) and compare and contrast their fat content. Which types of fats are featured? How many grams of each? Then put together a short essay about their likely effects within the body.

WORDS TO UNDERSTAND

electrolytes—any of the ions (as of sodium or calcium) that in biological fluid regulate or affect most metabolic processes (such as the flow of nutrients into and waste products out of cells)

hypertonic—the state of containing more osmotic pressure than another fluid, especially intra/extracellular fluid

hyponatremia—a condition in which the sodium concentration in blood is too low (less than 135 mmol/liter)

tonicity—a measure of the concentration of an environment and how it moves across a membrane

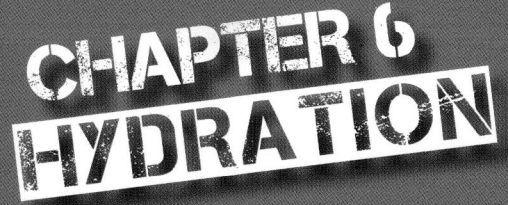

CHAPTER 6
HYDRATION

DEFINITION OF HYDRATION

Cells are made up mostly of water, including but not limited to muscle cells, brain cells, and blood cells. Experts say that up to 60 percent of our body is water. According to the *Journal of Biological Chemistry,* the brain and heart are 73 percent water, the lungs around 83 percent water, the skin up to 64 percent, muscles, kidneys, and other organs up to 79 percent water, and even bones contain 31 percent water. Outside of basic composition, water also acts as an essential ingredient in metabolic processes. No wonder water is so important for us!

How can you make sure you're getting enough water?

According to the National Academies of Sciences, Engineering, and Medicine, men need about 15.5 cups (3.7 liters) of fluids daily, while women need around 11.5 cups (2.7 liters) of fluids a day. However, another systematic review showed that plain water accounts for "up to 58 percent of total beverage intake, with great variability from 21 to 58 percent between countries. This number was increased to 51–75 percent in adolescents."

Water itself, however, isn't the only contributor to hydration. Maintaining fluid homeostasis requires a balance of water *and* salt content in the cells.

DEHYDRATION

To stay hydrated, we have to consider the **tonicity** of our cells in relation to their environment. Tonicity refers to the balance of water and salt in a concentrated solution. For example, isotonic solutions have an equal concentration of salt and water, such as for an intravenous saline drip. It's the same when the amount of water/salt within your cells equals the amount of water/salt outside of them.

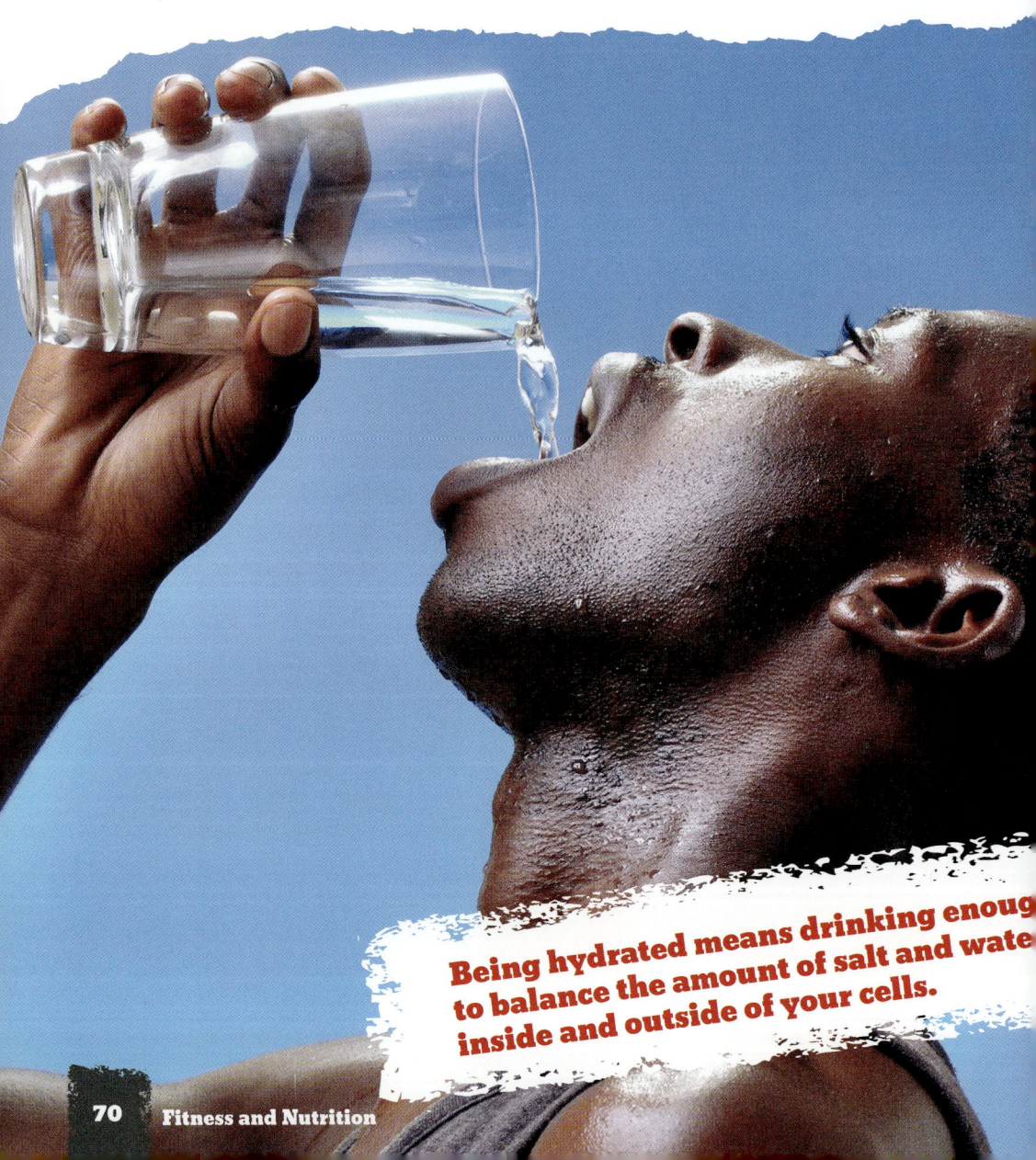

Being hydrated means drinking enough to balance the amount of salt and water inside and outside of your cells.

Exercise, breathing, and normal daily activity require water, so our cells are constantly asking for more. Fortunately, water (when available) naturally flows across the membrane and into the cell along a concentration gradient. That means that when salt concentration within the cell is higher compared to the outside, water will enter the cell in an attempt to equalize both concentrations.

However, this can only happen if water is available. When we don't drink enough water, the concentration outside of the cell remains low as well, restricting the natural flow. The conditions inside the cell become **hypertonic**. It might even cause more water to leave the cell, leading to dehydration.

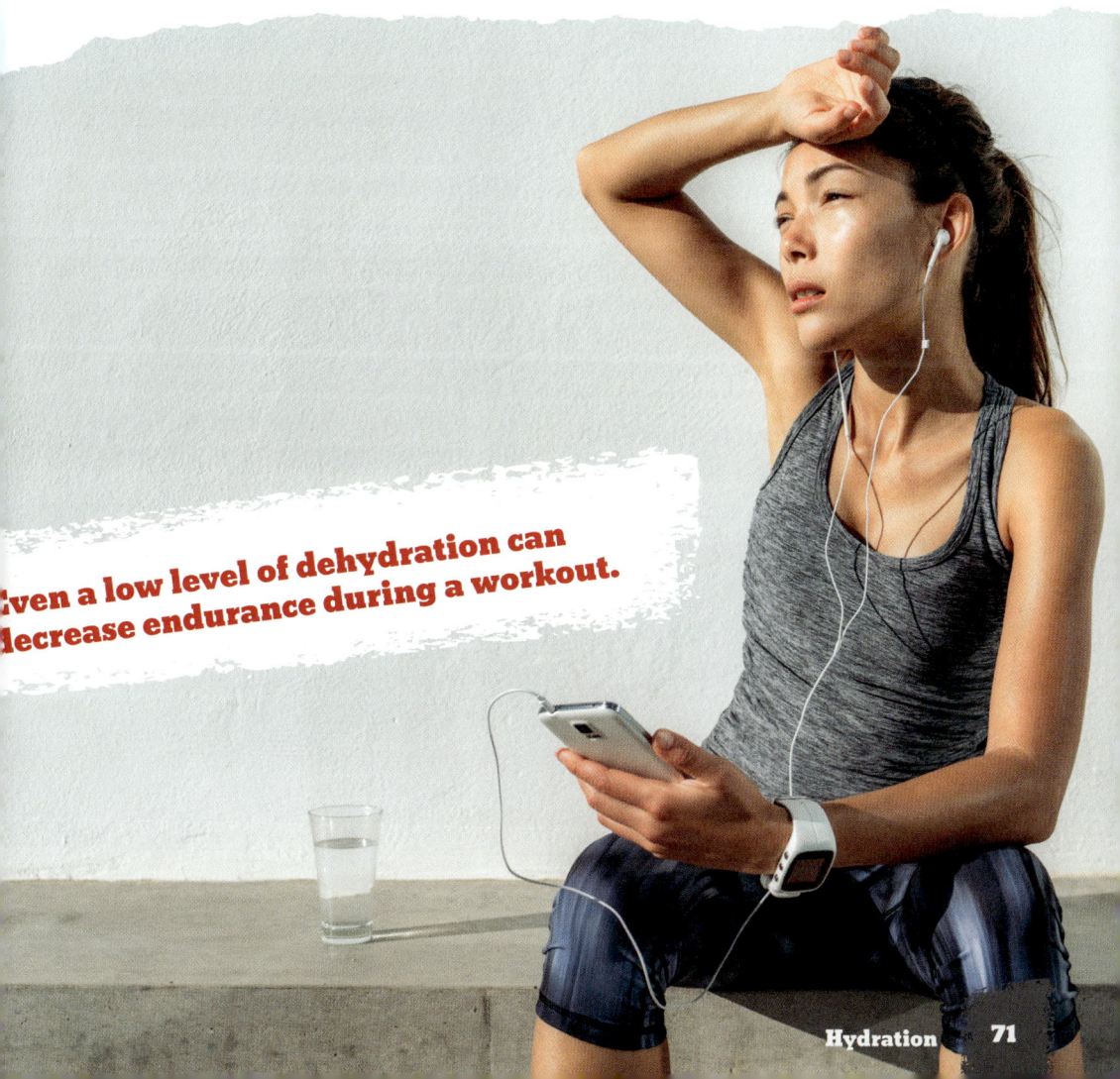

Even a low level of dehydration can decrease endurance during a workout.

If too much salt in the bloodstream can dehydrate us, then why do athletes need **electrolytes**?

Under extreme conditions, such as really hot temperatures or strenuous workouts, we lose salts through sweat. This decreases the overall concentration—both in AND outside of the cell. Electrolytes aren't just a part of maintaining cellular tonicity. They also help conduct electric currents, facilitate muscle contraction, and help metabolism. Athletes, in particular, need electrolytes, as sports rely on reaction time, energy, and muscular output. The American College of Sports Medicine, therefore, recommends including 0.5–0.7 g of sodium per gram of water to facilitate quick rehydration.

At its worst, dehydration can be extremely dangerous to the point of fatality. Even if you're nowhere near that extreme, a small level of dehydration can impact your physical and cognitive function. Your exercise endurance drops, you're less powerful, and it takes longer to recover. Dehydration reduces memory and recall, increases cognitive fog, and slows processing speeds. It can also just plain make you feel crummy. Therefore, in order to be at your best, try regularly drinking water and adding electrolytes to your intense workouts.

IS IT POSSIBLE TO DRINK TOO MUCH WATER?

Overhydration is possible, but rare outside of endurance sports. As previously mentioned, your cells require homeostasis to function properly. Too far in either direction and negative consequences arise. Severe sodium loss combined with overconsumption of water can lead to overhydration, also known as **hyponatremia**. Although it can be fatal if not treated, overhydration is very hard to cause. As long as you're eating an adequate amount of sodium and don't drink more than 0.8–1.0 liters per hour, you should be okay. However, if any symptoms start to arise, always consult a medical professional.

How much should active people drink? Check out the answers in this video.

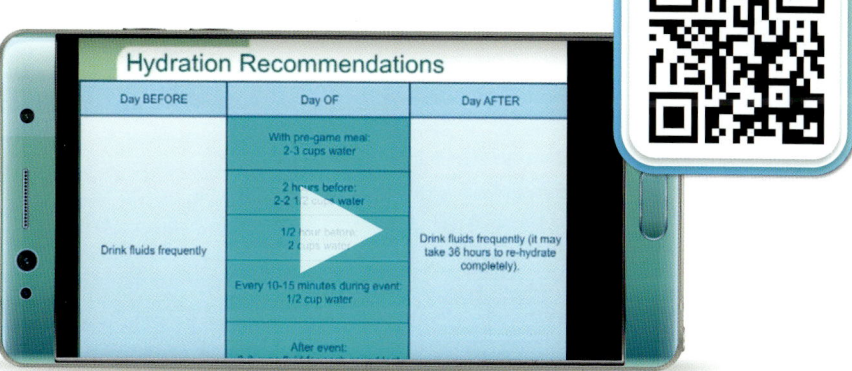

WHAT AND HOW MUCH TO DRINK

Throughout the day

According to *Medical News Today*, our kidneys (the organs responsible for urine elimination) can process up to 27–33 ounces of water per hour. Assuming you're eating, regular digestion will slow the distribution of water from the stomach. That's why if you chug a ton of water, you might feel bloated for a while. As food contains plenty of salts, the general recommendation is to stick to plain water throughout the day. Pop, electrolyte drinks, and even fruit juice all come with too much sugar. Unless you're in the middle of the state championship or hiking through the deserts of Arizona, it's wise to stick to plain water.

A recent report from the Institute of Medicine set overall guidelines for "women at approximately 2.7 liters (91 ounces) of total water—from all beverages and foods—each day, and men an average of approximately 3.7 liters (125 ounces daily) of total water."

Carrying a reusable water bottle to school, class, practice, or work will help you stay hydrated. You can even mark off your daily

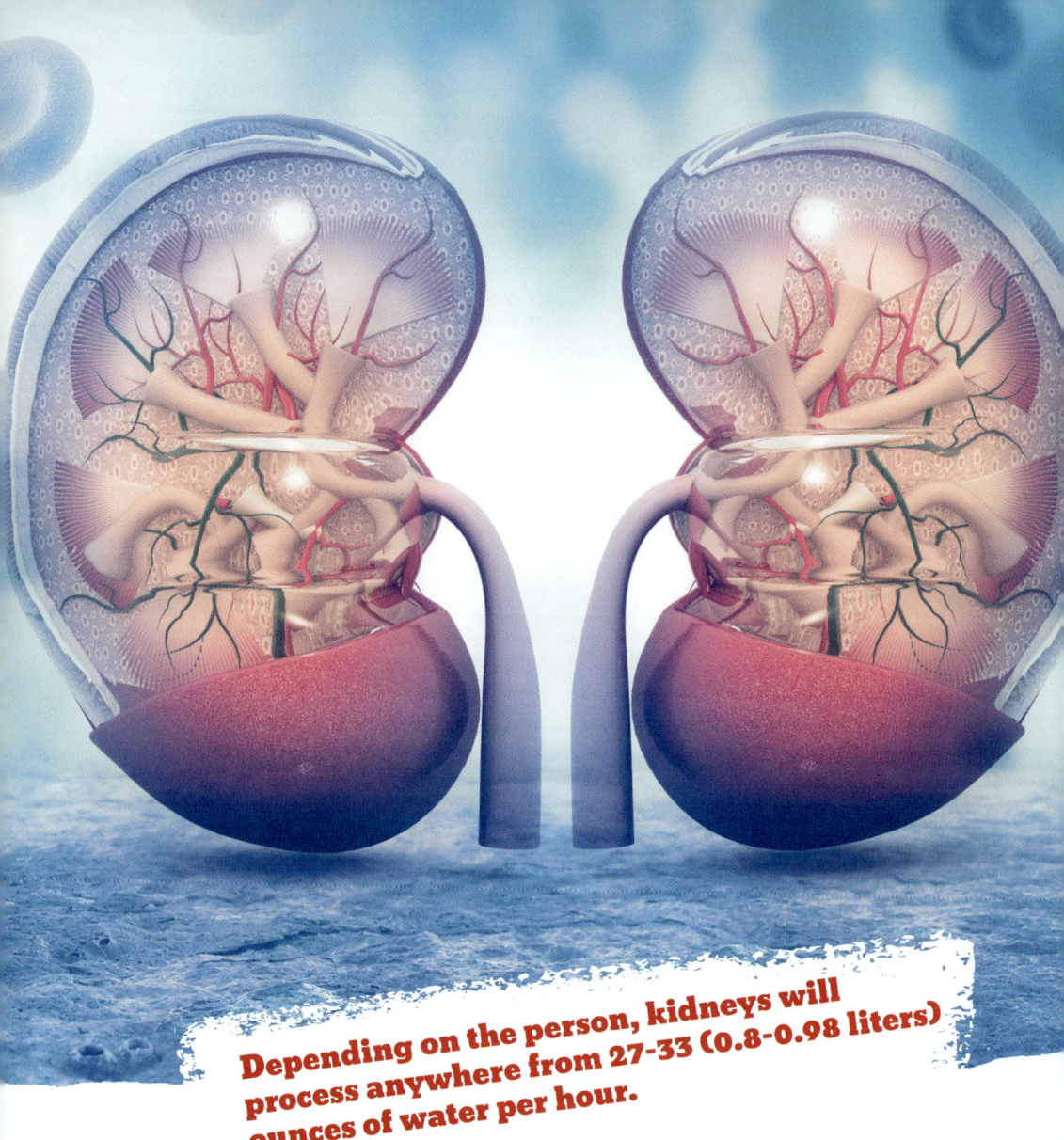

Depending on the person, kidneys will process anywhere from 27-33 (0.8-0.98 liters) ounces of water per hour.

target with a marker to stay on track. Consider keeping a personal hydration log by measuring the color of your urine throughout the day. It might sound gross, but it's the best objective indicator of your fluid concentration. The darker your urine, the more dehydrated you are. However you measure it, make sure you're sipping water regularly throughout the day.

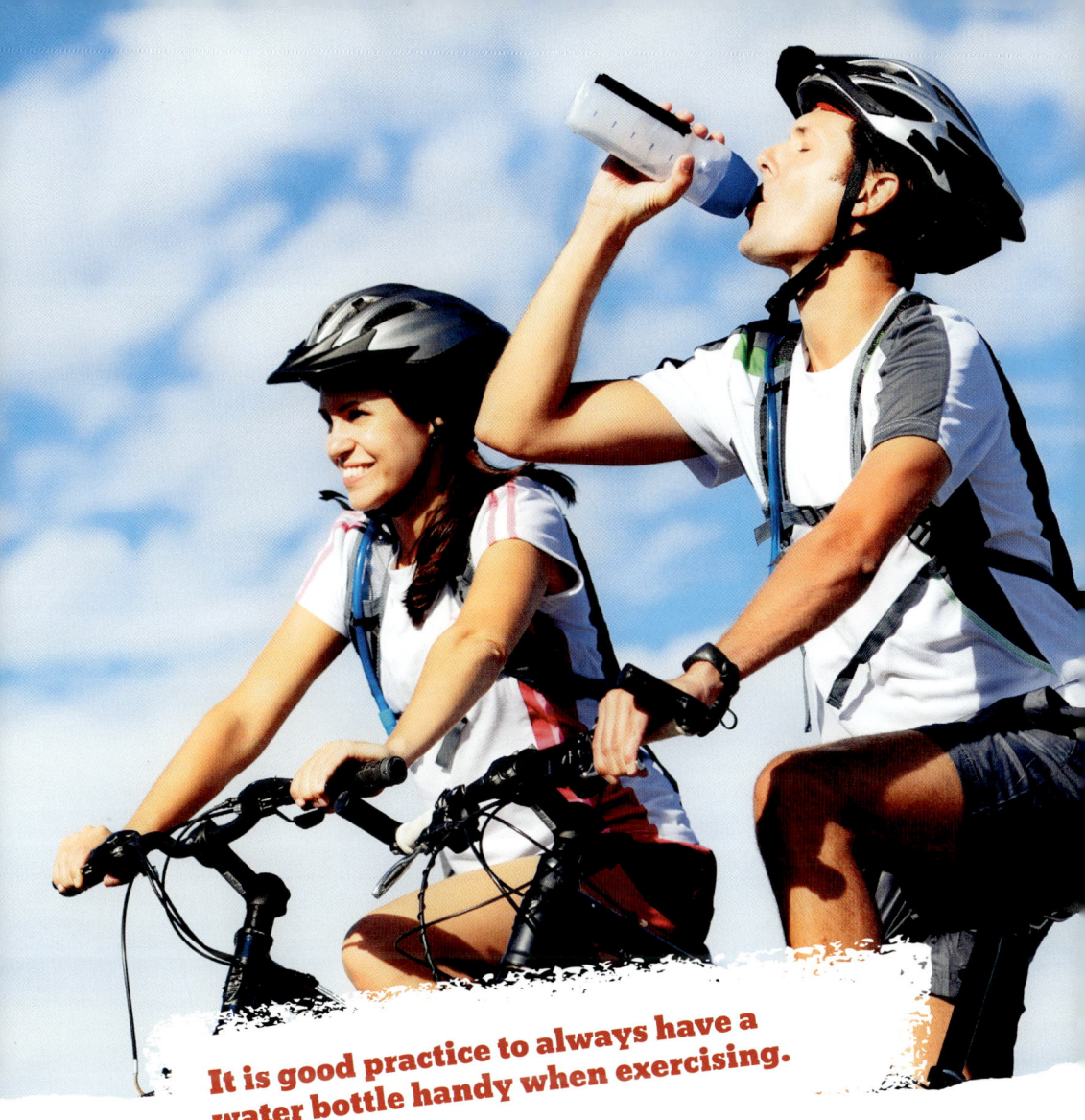

It is good practice to always have a water bottle handy when exercising.

Around workouts

In addition to the aforementioned guidelines around sodium intake, drink 500–600 ml of water 3 hours before exercise. Add 200–300 ml every 20–30 minutes for activities longer than an hour, especially in the hot sun. Always keep a water bottle on hand to increase the chance of consistent intake.

People do lose weight immediately after strenuous exercise, but that is primarily due to losing water.

To get a more objective measure, athletes can measure their pre-/post-training weight. No—this isn't an indication of actual fat loss. Rather, the more fluid mass we lose from sweat and breathing, the lighter our bodies become. Every pound of weight lost in practice or even overnight represents 16–24 ounces of fluid loss. Taking body weight pre- and post-training lets the athlete know how much water was lost, so it is a valuable tool in fluid replenishment.

TEXT-DEPENDENT QUESTIONS

1. Identify and define two objective measurements of hydration that you can use throughout the day.

2. What is tonicity, and what does it have to do with hydration?

3. What additional hydration recommendations exist for athletes or those doing intense exercise?

RESEARCH PROJECT

Sports drinks have become commonplace among athletic events today, but they didn't always exist. Research the history of carbohydrate–electrolyte mixed sports drinks. When and why were they invented? How have they evolved? Put together a short PowerPoint or other visual presentation on the topic.

WORDS TO UNDERSTAND

fibrous—containing, consisting of, or resembling fibers
manipulation—to manage or utilize skillfully
thermodynamics—the science concerned with the relations between heat and mechanical energy or work, and the conversion of one into the other

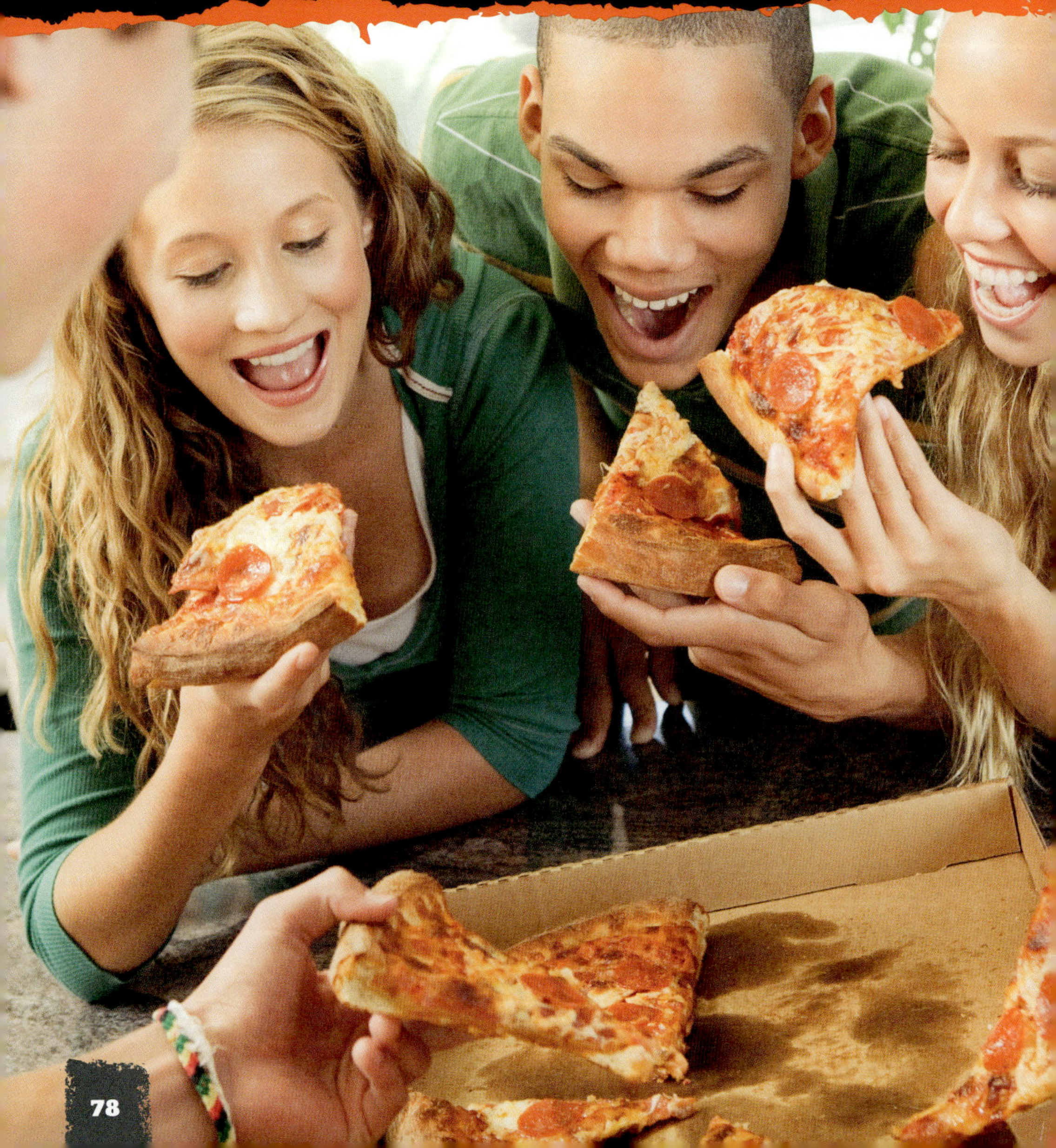

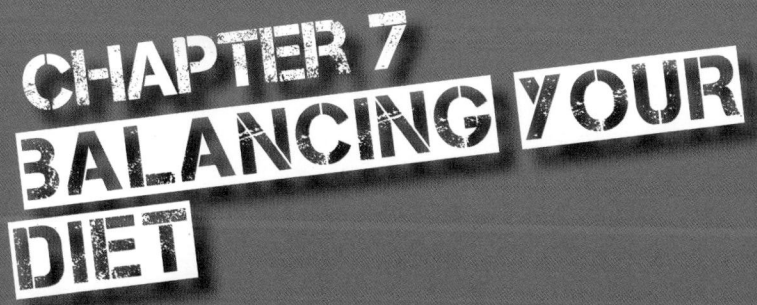

CHAPTER 7
BALANCING YOUR DIET

WHEN AND HOW MUCH OF WHAT SHOULD WE EAT?

Due to developmental needs, adolescents require more food than most other age groups. A lot is going on in your body as a teenager, and you're quite literally building yourself into an adult. As you'll remember from earlier chapters, the food you consume lays the groundwork for physical structures, immune function, neural capacity, and more. Here are some general guidelines for you to follow:

Focus on nutrient-dense foods

Fat loss (and maintenance) follows the simple law of **thermodynamics**— you need fewer calories in than out to lose fat, and a relatively equal amount to maintain. Your stomach is not a calorie counter, it's a volume counter. Dense foods, like fruit and vegetables, fill you up while limiting calories. On the flip side, high-calorie, low-density foods leave you not only hungry and craving more, but they add empty calories.

In that same vein...

Don't drink your calories!

One of the easiest, most common ways to butcher your healthy lifestyle comes in liquid form. Whether it's a sugary coffee, your favorite pop, or fruit juice, calorie-heavy drinks do nothing for you. They might taste delicious, but inside, your body stores those calories without feeling satiated. In fact, you'll probably crave more.

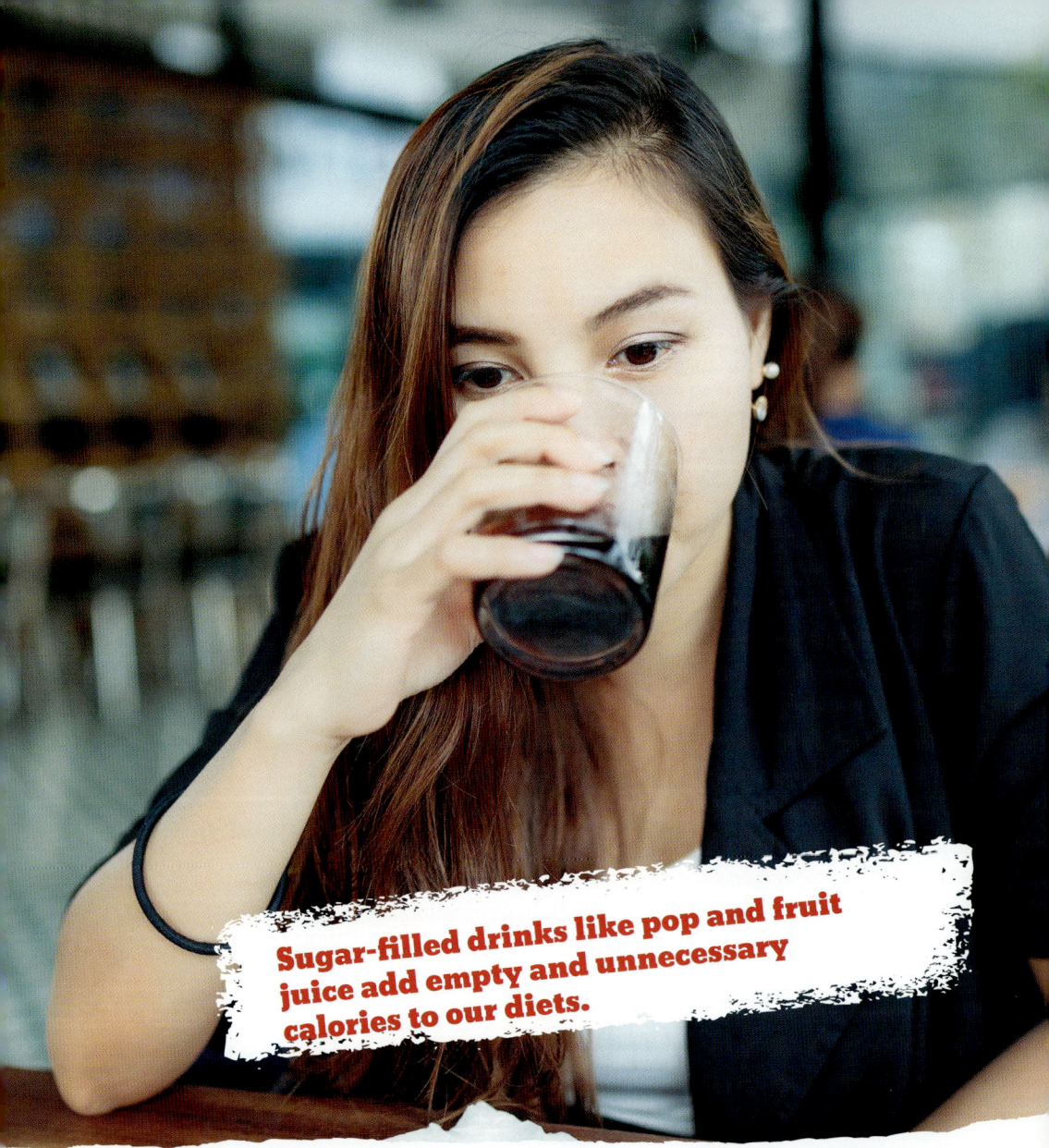

Sugar-filled drinks like pop and fruit juice add empty and unnecessary calories to our diets.

Since it barely registers those drinks as food, your body will demand you eat a normal diet on top of it. In your 10-minute coffee run, you've added 500 empty calories. No matter how healthy the rest of your day is, you can't get those back. Sure, you could skip a meal, but that leaves you miserable, hungry, and dissatisfied. Again, this is the challenge with healthy eating we're trying to overcome.

The link between protein and building muscle mass is examined in this video.

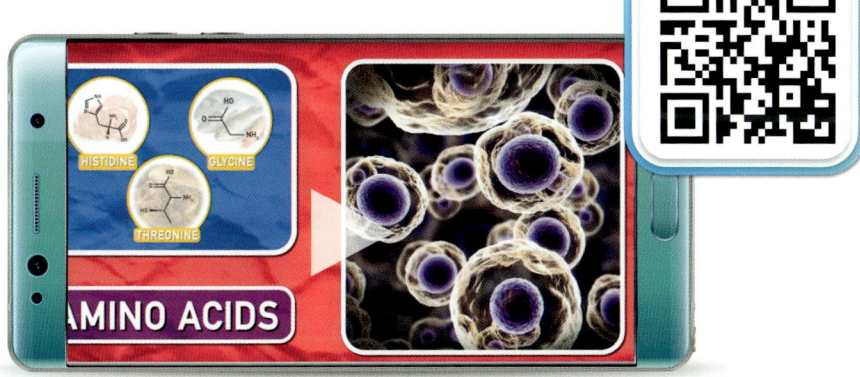

Other macronutrient considerations

You can't go anywhere without someone demonizing a macronutrient. All carbs are bad. Don't eat fatty foods. While neither of these is true, protein rarely comes under fire. That is because lean proteins are the core of any healthy diet.

Protein is the macronutrient responsible for muscle growth, cellular repair, connective tissue health, and plenty of other bodily processes. It's also the macronutrient that fills us up the most. When controlling for total calorie content, research shows that protein curbs hunger better than fats or carbs. Something that puts on muscle, protects our bones, and helps us eat less? That's a recipe for good health.

When looking at a nutritious meal, your general template could be:

- Your protein of choice
- A nutrient-dense carb/fat of choice (i.e., sweet potato, rice, avocado, nuts, etc.)
- Vegetables for micronutrients

Specific goals require a bit more macronutrient **manipulation** based on activity level and body type. For general purposes, focus on lean protein, nutrient-dense foods, and a plate full of veggies.

NUTRIENT TIMING

You don't have to eat three square meals every day for good nutrition. Nor do you need to snack 10 times (or even eat breakfast!).

Of course, most of these commonly cited recommendations come with some truth. Eating frequently can help curb hunger. Breakfast tends to start us off on a good foot, especially if you've got a long day of school ahead of you. You'll want some fuel to activate your brain in the morning that can sustain you until lunch. If it's the summer, however, techniques such as intermittent fasting have been shown to control hunger hormones and weight gain in adults. Before you start manipulating your diet, always meet with a physician so they can check if it's safe or even recommended for your age, height, and body type.

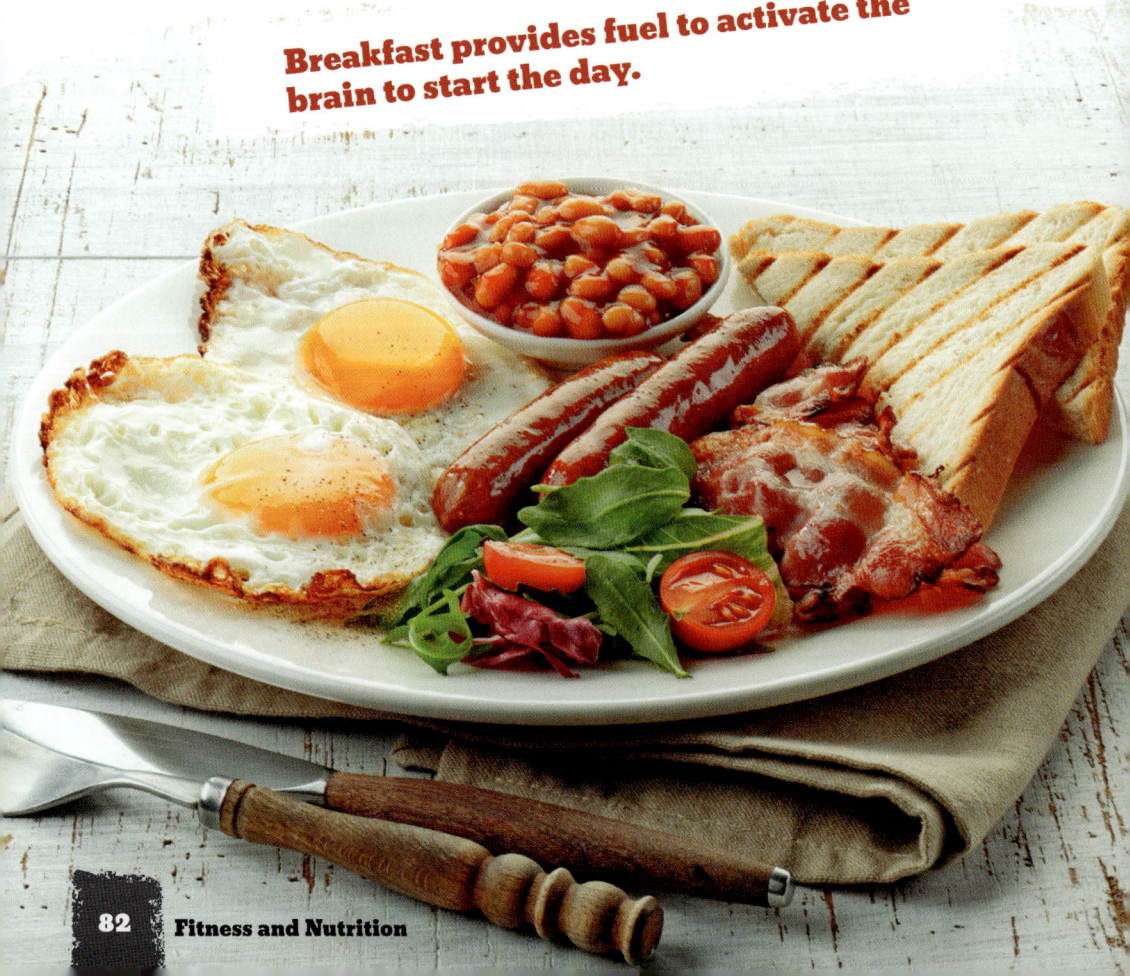

Breakfast provides fuel to activate the brain to start the day.

Below are a few recommendations for healthy eating. Remember—there are no hard-and-fast rules. The most important thing is to develop a positive relationship with food so that it can fuel your growth and development.

When to eat carbs

- Try to primarily eat **fibrous**, non-processed, natural foods
- Choose simple sugars 30 minutes before or after an intense workout, possibly during a long event; otherwise, use sparingly
- Choose low-glycemic carbs at meals, unless it's just before a training session
- Eat more carbs if you're incredibly active, less if you're very sedentary

When to eat fats

- Aim for primarily monounsaturated and polyunsaturated fats
- Avoid fats around your workouts, unless it's a very low-intensity session, such as a walk
- Eating good fats before bed can help facilitate overnight recovery
- Add about 30–60 ml (1–2 ounces) of fat to each meal

When to eat protein

- Shoot for 20 g of lean protein at every meal
- Add another 20 g after your workout to facilitate muscle growth
- Protein before bed can help you recover from muscular damage or physical stress
- Everyone needs protein! People with more mass will need more protein

HOW OFTEN SHOULD YOU EAT?

There's an assumption going around that eating more often increases your metabolism. In short, it doesn't really. Refer back to Chapter 2 for

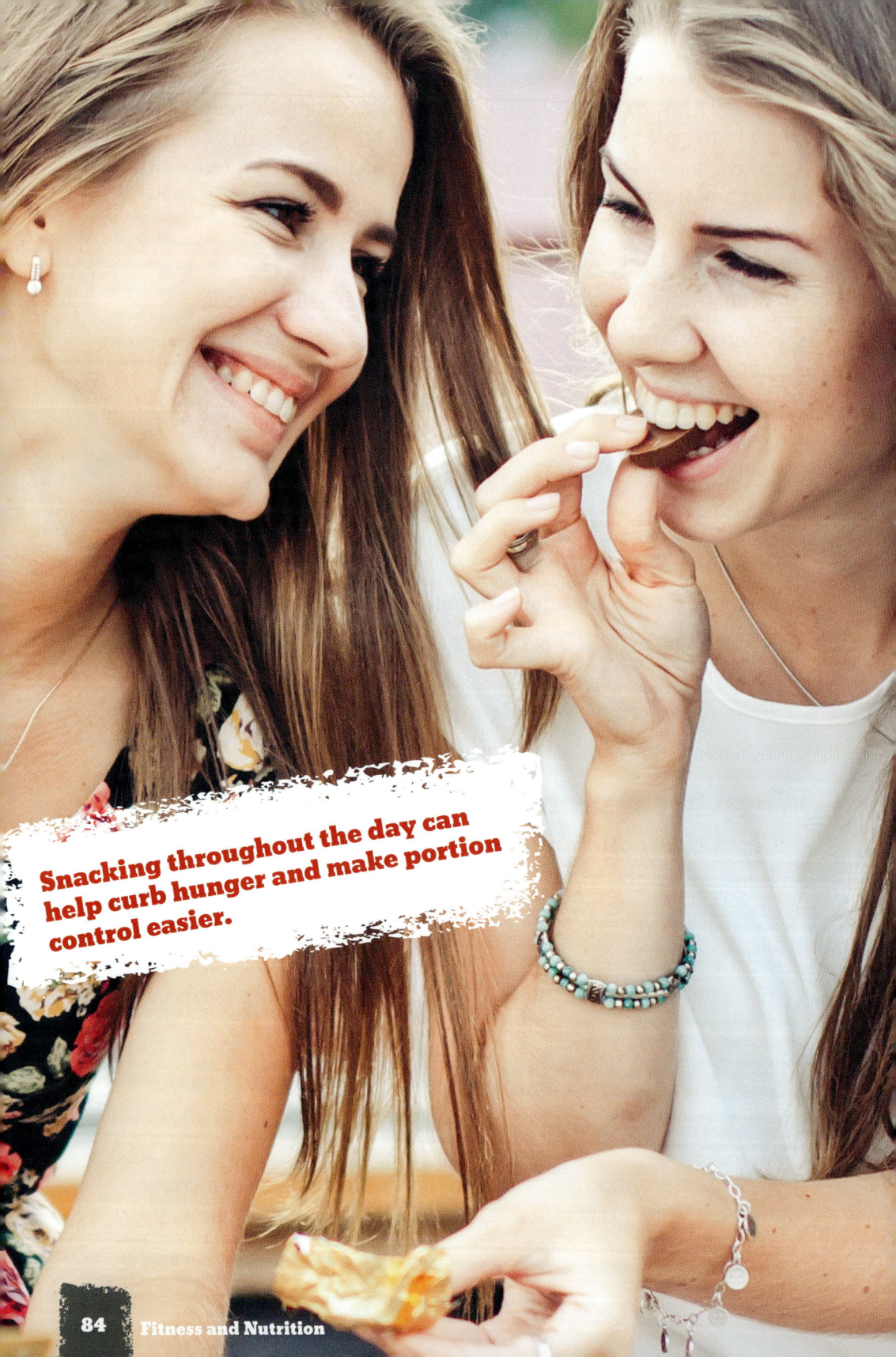

Snacking throughout the day can help curb hunger and make portion control easier.

the primary factors affecting your metabolic rate. Instead, eating more often can help with portion control and hunger, which ultimately tends to promote healthy eating habits.

For example, modern lifestyles present us with few opportunities to eat meals naturally during the day. We're rushed in the morning trying to get our day going. After fasting all night, we barely eat anything. Then lunch is a quick version of whatever's at the cafeteria, the fast-food restaurant, or what we had time to throw in a bag. Thanks to school and extracurriculars, it can be difficult to eat anything substantial until 7 or 8 pm—upon which we stuff our faces because we're so hungry.

If that sounds familiar, you're not alone. It just means all of our calories are centered on a time when we don't really need to fuel activity—a.k.a. during sleep. However, you can absolutely just spread your food out between three square meals. Another popular option is intermittent fasting, where you choose a certain amount of hours in the day to consolidate your meals. The right diet for you is one that fits your schedule, you can enjoy consistently, and keeps you healthy and happy.

Below is an example of what an eating schedule would look like for a high school athlete:

Breakfast, 6:30 am: Two eggs, bacon, and toast

Snack, 9 am: Low-fat yogurt with granola and nuts

Lunch, 11:30 am: Chicken breast, roasted sweet potato, and asparagus with olive oil

After school/pre-practice snack, 3 pm: 20 g whey protein shake blended with berries and oats

Post-workout shake, 5:30 pm: 20 g whey protein shake blended with berries and oats

Dinner, 7:30 pm: Steak, brown rice, and zucchini roasted with olive oil

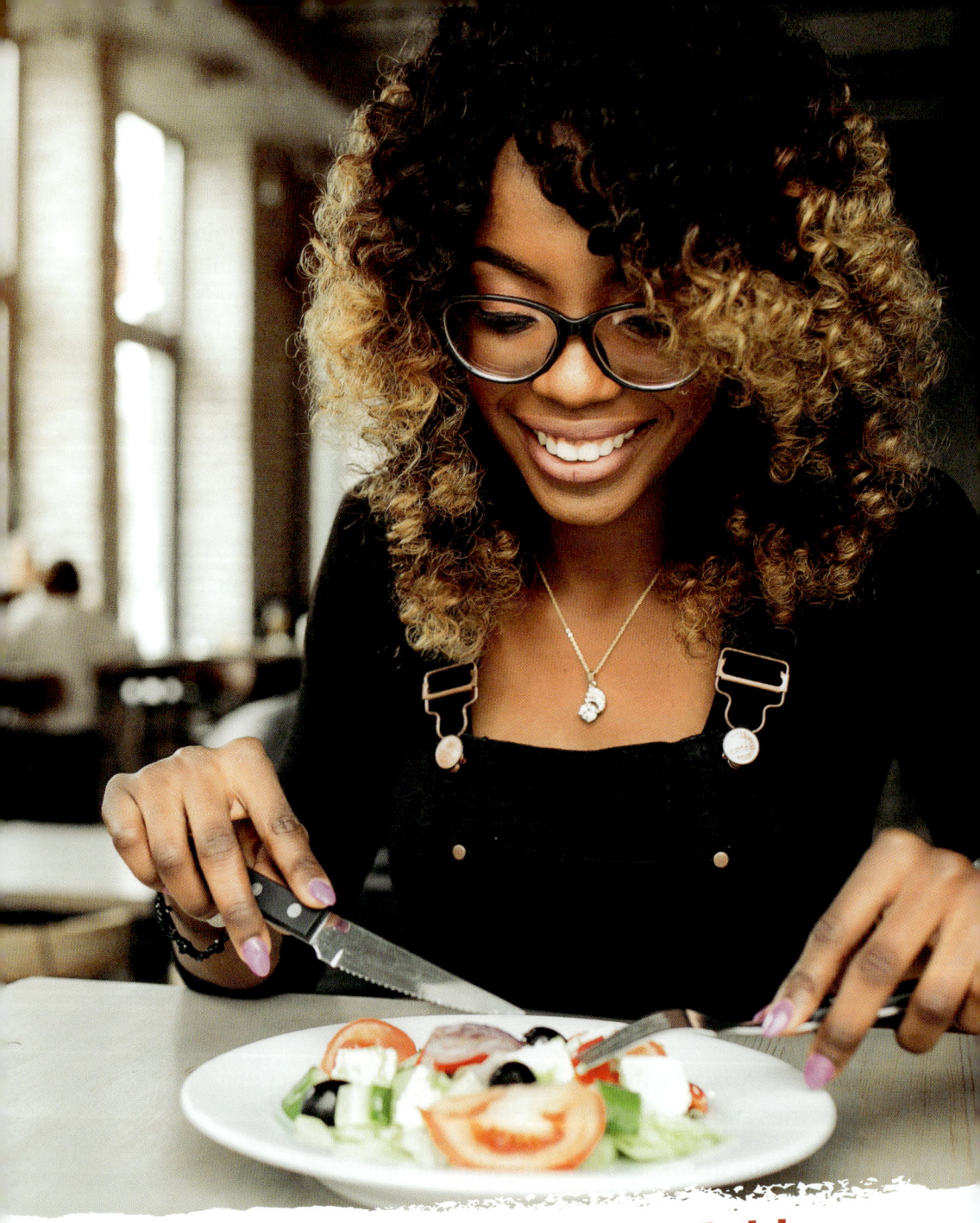

It is not always possible to schedule every meal, but you should try and eat well when the opportunity arises.

The above is simply an example. Your meals will vary depending on your schedule, resources, activity level, and likes and dislikes. Maybe you can't eat a snack during class, and that's okay! Just eat a bigger breakfast and lunch. Or maybe you don't play sports after school, and are involved in clubs, have a job, play video games, or just do homework instead. Whatever your schedule, you can adjust.

BUILDING MUSCLE VS. LOSING FAT. IS IT SIMPLY WEIGHTS VS. CARDIO?

Unless you have insane genetics (and are a teenage boy), you likely won't build muscle without lifting weights. You could develop lean muscle by doing non-traditional resistance training, such as running

EATING TO BE "FIT" VS. LOOKING FIT AESTHETICALLY—WHAT'S HEALTHY?

Important note: Aesthetics can be misleading, and body positivity is something to be celebrated. If you have ANY concerns about your mental, physical, or emotional health, or your relationship with food, always consult a professional. At the end of this book, you'll find a link to the Healthy Teen Project. Feel free to check it out whether you could use help, want guidance, or are simply curious or confused.

Healthy weight, body type, and aesthetics all vary from person to person. There's no universal "right" way to look. Instead of focusing on looking "fit," focus on healthy habits and a positive relationship with food and exercise. Get active and use food as fuel for your favorite pastimes. There are certain foods, however, that are bad for your health. Refer back to previous chapters for foods to eat sparingly. Healthy eating is about how your body feels more than it looks, especially as a teenager. Regardless, make sure you're getting your annual check-up with a physician, and consult with a dietician if any concerns arise.

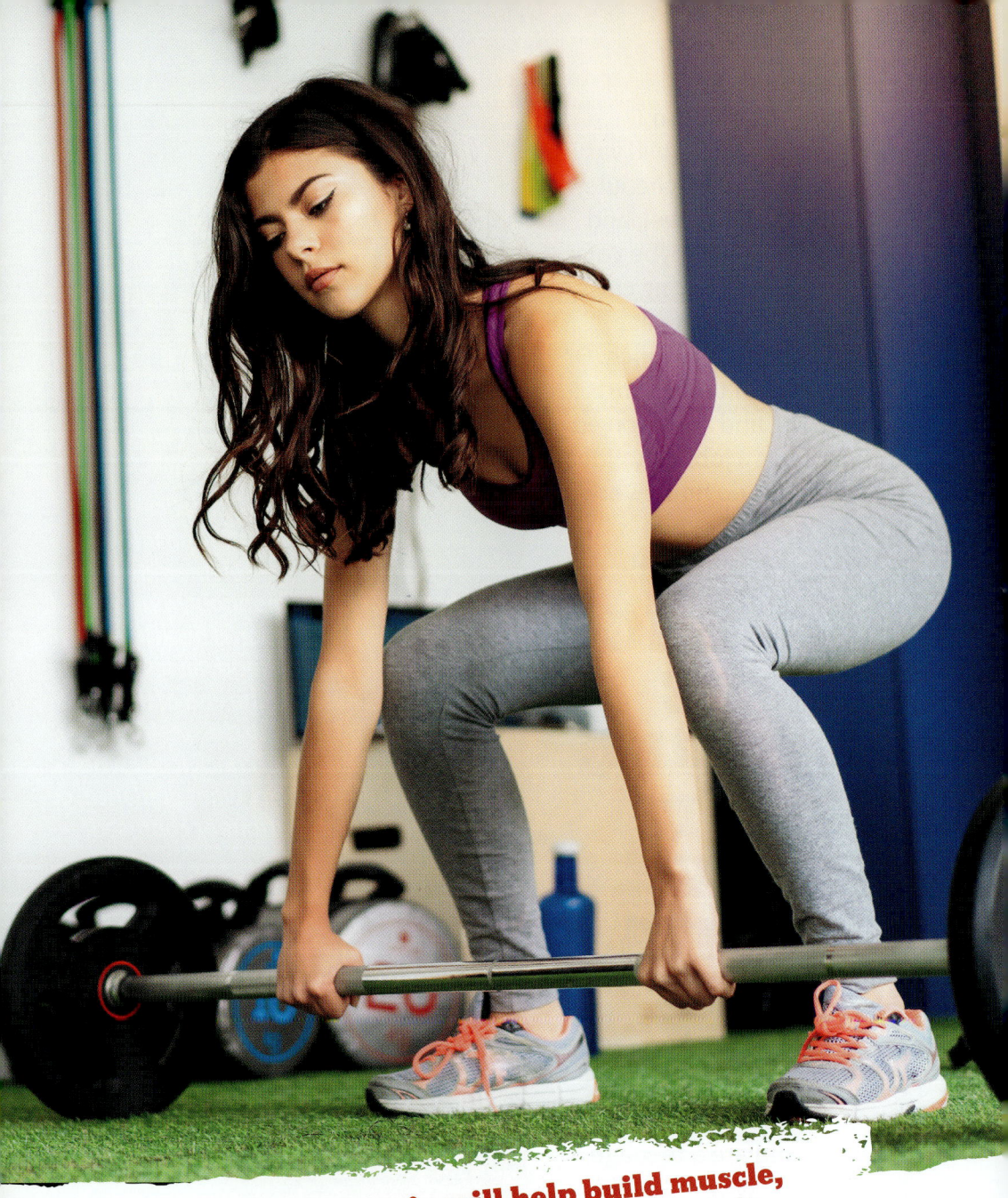

Eating protein will help build muscle, but only if a muscle-building activity goes along with it.

hills or bouldering. But in order to stimulate muscle-specific protein synthesis, you need that stimulus. Otherwise, all of those extra calories will just be stored as fat or burned off during cardio. The body adapts according to its demands. Therefore, if you're only doing cardio, it will assume you need your nutrients to fuel that. If you're not doing anything, it'll store them for some future emergency (such as hibernation, if you were a bear).

As a suggested guideline, here are some ways to adjust your daily intake to meet your fitness goals:

Daily caloric intake

Goal: Weight gain

Heavy training days: 20–22 times body weight

Light training days: 18–20 times body weight

Goal: Maintenance

Heavy training days: 16–18 times body weight

Light training days: 14–16 times body weight

Goal: Weight loss

Heavy training days: 14–16 times body weight

Light training days: 12–14 times body weight

Calories per macronutrient

Protein: 4 calories per gram

Carbohydrate: 4 calories per gram

Fat: 9 calories per gram

Macronutrient intake breakdown by body type

Ectomorphs (naturally thin with skinny limbs)—25 percent protein, 55 percent carbohydrate, 20 percent fat

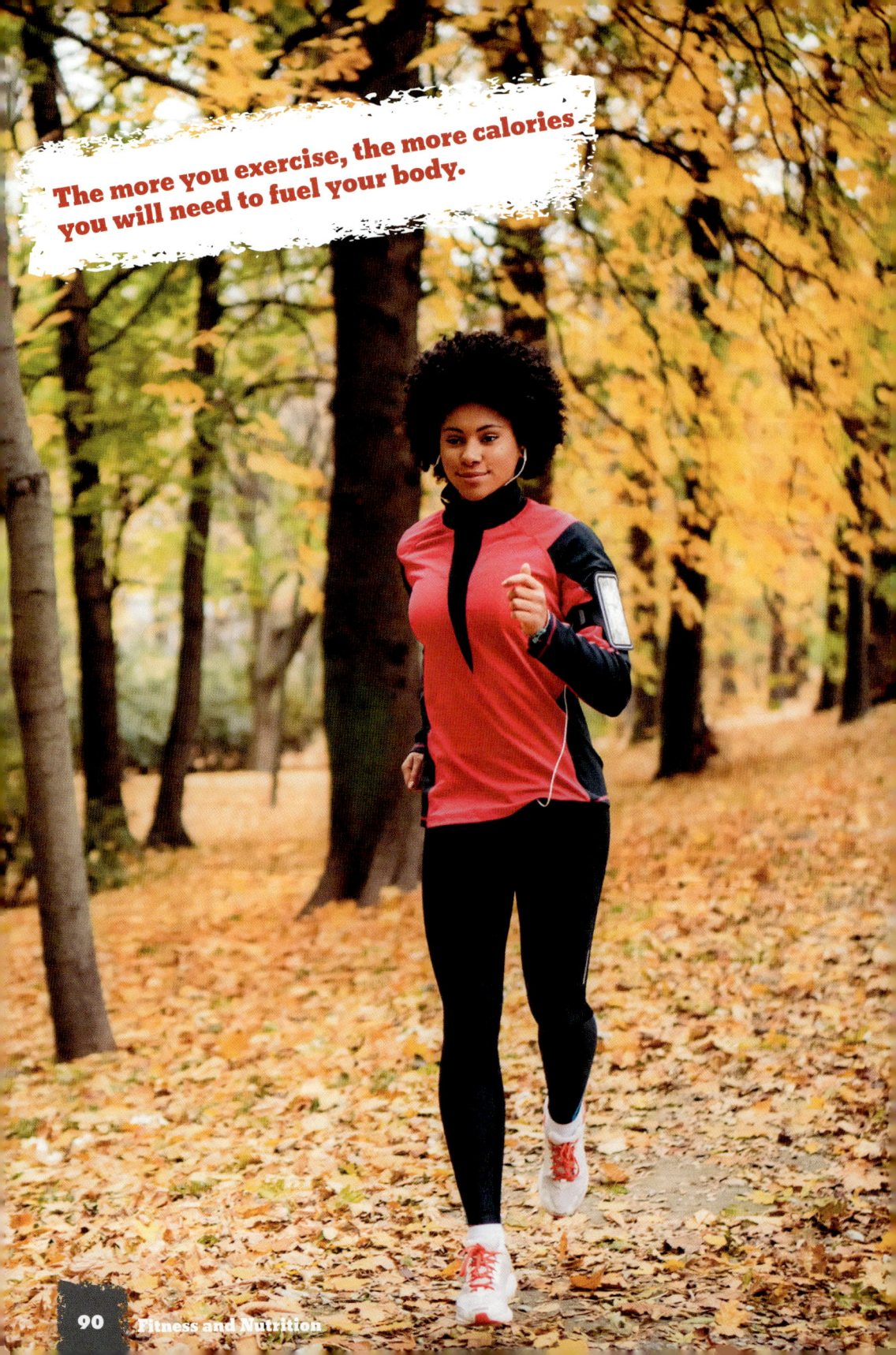

Mesomorphs (naturally muscular/athletic)—30 percent protein, 40 percent carbohydrate, 30 percent fat

Endomorphs (naturally broad and thick)—35 percent protein, 25 percent carbohydrate, 40 percent fat

TEXT-DEPENDENT QUESTIONS

1. How can you manipulate your macronutrient intake based on your fitness goals and activity level?

2. How does nutrient timing play a role in nutrition, and does it affect your metabolism?

3. Name three healthy habits around nutrition, and how you can implement them in your daily life.

RESEARCH PROJECT

Research to design a suggested weekly meal plan for yourself, a friend, or a family member using the information you learned about them. Make sure to include their schedule, activity level, age, height and weight, and fitness goals.

SERIES GLOSSARY OF KEY TERMS

Cardiorespiratory – of or relating to the heart and the respiratory system.

Circuit training – a workout technique involving a series of exercises performed in rotation with minimal rest, often using different pieces of apparatus.

Fatigue – weariness or exhaustion from labor, exertion, or stress.

HDL cholesterol – also known as good cholesterol. A lipoprotein of blood plasma that is composed of a high proportion of protein with little triglyceride and cholesterol and that is correlated with reduced risk of atherosclerosis.

Hormone – a product of living cells that circulates in body fluids (such as blood) and produces a specific and often stimulatory effect on the activity of cells, usually remote from its point of origin.

Lactic acid – a normally present hygroscopic organic acid ($C_3H_6O_3$), especially in muscle tissue, that is a by-product of anaerobic glycolysis, produced in carbohydrate matter usually by bacterial fermentation, and used especially in food and medicine and in industry.

LDL cholesterol – also known as bad cholesterol. A lipoprotein of blood plasma that is composed of a moderate proportion of protein with little triglyceride and a high proportion of cholesterol and that is associated with increased probability of developing atherosclerosis.

Metabolism – the chemical changes in living cells by which energy is provided for vital processes and activities, and new material is assimilated.

Micronutrients – a chemical element or substance (such as calcium or vitamin C) that is essential in minute amounts to the growth and health of a living organism.

Modification – the making of a limited change in something, such as an exercise, that makes the exercise easier.

Physiology – a branch of biology that deals with the functions and activities of life or of living matter (such as organs, tissues, or cells) and of the physical and chemical phenomena involved.

Resistance – of, relating to, or being an exercise involving pushing or pulling against the source of an opposing force (such as a weight) to increase strength.

Tempo – rate of motion or activity.

FURTHER READING

Benardot, D. *Advanced Sports Nutrition*. Champaign: Human Kinetics, 2020.

Bjorn, Nicholas. *Fitness Nutrition: The Ultimate Fitness Guide*. Scotts Valley: CreateSpace, 2015.

Flanagan, Shalane, and Elyse Kopecky. *Run Fast. Eat Slow: Recipes for Athletes*. New York: Rodale Fitness, 2016.

Gundry, Steven. *The Plant Paradox: The Hidden Dangers in Healthy Foods That Cause Disease and Weight Gain*. New York: Harper Collins, 2017.

INTERNET RESOURCES

http://www.healthyteenproject.com/resources-ca

The Healthy Teen Project provides help and assistance to teens who may be dealing with eating-related issues, featuring experts in the field and nationally recognized resources.

https://www.girlshealth.gov/nutrition

Girls Health showcases common health concerns faced by young women today, including nutrition, fitness, disability, relationships, bullying, and more.

https://www.precisionnutrition.com

Precision Nutrition is an internationally recognized resource for evidence-based information around fitness and exercise.

https://www.teamusa.org/nutrition

The U.S. Olympic Committee shares advice from its expert nutritionists on how to eat well to fuel athletic performance.

https://renaissanceperiodization.com/expert-advice

Renaissance Periodization collects advice from dieticians, PhD's, and sports performance coaches on how to eat well around strength training to reach specific goals.

INDEX

A
Adenosine triphosphate (ATP), 32, 36
Adipose tissue, 57, 63
Aerobic metabolism, 38
Aesthetics, 87
Age, and metabolism, 26
Alanine, 47, 48
American College of Sports Medicine, 72
American Heart Association, 61
American Journal of Clinical Nutrition, 61
Amino acids, 43
    essential, 44–46
    non-essential, 47–50
Anabolic processes, 44
Annals of Internal Medicine, 11
Appetite, reduction of, 52–54
Archives of Internal Medicine, 38
Arginine, 48, 54
Asparagine, 48
Aspartic acid, 48
Athletes
    carbs for, 38, 40–41
    eating schedule for, 85
    measuring their pre-/post-training weight, 77
Atkins, Robert, 34
Atkins diet, 34
Avocado, 59

B
Bad fats, 61–64
Balanced diet, 11–13, 39, 79
Basal metabolic rate (BMR), 22
"Blue Zones," 15–17
Body fat, 57
Brain function, 58–60
Branched-chain amino acids (BCAAs), 44, 52
Breakfast, 82
British Medical Journal, 63
Burning calories, 22–24

C
Caloric density, 21
Calories, 19, 79–80
    burning, 22–24
    daily requirements, 21–22, 89
    low-calorie diets, 34
    per macronutrient, 89
    measuring, 19–22
    metabolism and, 24–28
    overconsumption of, 64
    tracking consumption of, 20–21
Canadian Family Physician, 12
Carbohydrates (carbs), 9, 31, 54
    for athletes, 38, 40–41
    benefits of, 31
    and fats, 63
    intake recommendations, 83
    for non-athletes, 38
Cell membranes, 58
Chronic inflammation, 60–61
Complex carbs, 31
Cortisol, 60–61
Cysteine, 48

D
Daily calorie requirements, 21–22, 89
Daily water intake, 69, 73
Dehydration, 70–72
Dense foods, 79
Department of Health and Human Services, 13
Dietary carbs, 31
Dietary fats, 57
    types of, 57
Dietary protein, benefits of
    increased muscle mass, 52
    injury repair, 54
    reduced appetite, 52–54
Diets, 61
    balancing, 79–91
    and health, 11–15, 39, 43
    measuring calories in, 19–22
    plant-based, 52
Disaccharides, 31
Docosahexaenoic acid (DHA), 58

E
Eating schedule (example), for high school athlete, 85
Ectomorphs, 89
80 percent rule, following, 17
Electrolytes, 72
Endomorphs, 91
Endurance exercise, 10
Essential amino acids, 44–46
Eustress, 7
Exercise, 7
    balanced diet and, 11–13
    burning calories, 24
    food consumption and, 9–10
    water intake during, 75–77
Exercise-free life, cases of, 12

F
Fats, 9, 54, 57
    bad, 61–64
    calories consumption, 64
    carbs and, 63
    daily intake, 66
    dietary, 57
    good, 58–61
    intake recommendations, 83
Fitness
    diet/exercise, as essential to, 13–15
    goals, 89
    vs. health, 7–8
Food consumption, 9–10, 79

G
Glucose, 32, 33
Glutamic acid, 50
Glutamine, 50, 54
Glycemic index, 33
Glycine, 50
Glycogen, 64–65
Glycolysis, 38
Good fats, 58–61
    brain function and, 58–60
    building cell membranes, 58
    reducing inflammation, 60–61
Gut health, 28

H
Harvard Health, 43
Health
    defined, 7
    diet and, 11–15
    fitness and, 7–8
    nutrition and, 9

Health.gov, 21
Healthy eating
   habits, promoting, 85, 87
   recommendations for, 83
Histidine, 45
Homeostasis, 9
Hormones, 26
Hydration
   definition of, 69
   recommendations, 73
Hydrogenation, 63
Hyponatremia, 72

I
Inactivity, risk of, 11–12
Inflammation, 60–61
Injury repair, 54
Institute of Medicine, 73
Insulin, 26, 33
Insulin resistance, 33
Intermittent fasting, 82, 85
Isoleucine, 45, 47

J
Journal of Biological Chemistry, 69

K
Ketogenic (keto) diet, 34–35, 54
Ketosis, 34
Kidneys, process of, 73
Kilocalorie, 19

L
Leucine, 45, 52
Low-carb dieting, 34, 38
Lysine, 45–46

M
Macronutrient considerations, 81, 89
Medical News Today, 73
Mediterranean diet, 58
Medium-chain triglycerides, 61
Mesomorphs, 91
Metabolic equivalent of a task (MET), 24
Metabolism, 24–28, 54
Methionine, 46, 47
Micronutrients, 9, 38

Mitochondria, 22, 25
Monosaccharides, 31
Monounsaturated fats, 57, 58
Movement, importance of, 11–12
mTOR pathway, 52
Muscle mass
   increased, 52
   lean, 26, 87–89
   protein and, 81, 88

N
National Academies of Sciences, Engineering, and Medicine, 69
"Net carbs," 34
Non-athletes, carbs for, 38, 40–41
Non-essential amino acids, 47–50
Nutrient-dense foods, 79
Nutrient timing, 82–83
Nutrition, 9
Nuts, 47

O
Okinawa, Japan, 16
Omega-3 fatty acid, 58
Overhydration, 72

P
Paleo diet, 54
PDCAAS (protein digestibility-corrected amino acid scores), 55
Peterman, Mynie, 34
Phenylalanine, 46, 47
Physical fitness, defined, 8
Plant-based diets, 52
Polysaccharides, 31
Polyunsaturated fats, 57, 58
Proline, 50
Protein-rich foods, 9–10
Proteins, 43
   benefits of dietary protein, 52–54
   daily allowance of, 43
   eating, 88
   essential amino acids, 44–46
   intake recommendations, 83
   lean, 81

   non-essential amino acids, 47–50
   overeating, 54–55
   in plant-based diets, 52

R
Respiratory exchange ratio (RER), 36
Resting metabolic rate (RMR), 24

S
Saturated fats, 57, 61–63
Seafood, 49
Sedentary lifestyles, symptoms and side effects of, 12–13
Serine, 50
Stress relief, 8
Sugar, 64–65

T
Testosterone, 26, 27
Thermodynamics, 79
Threonine, 46
Tonicity, 70
Trail mix, 66
Trans fats, 63–64
Triglycerides, 61, 63
Tryptophan, 46
Tyrosine, 50, 51

U
Undereating, risks of, 11
University of Bristol, 11
U.S. Department of Health and Human Services, 8

V
Valine, 46
Vitamins and minerals, need for, 9

W
Water
   body and, 69
   intake, 69
      throughout the day, 73–74
      around workouts, 75–77
   overconsumption of, 72

AUTHOR BIOGRAPHY

Kimber Rozier is a NSCA certified strength and conditioning specialist who holds dual Bachelor's degrees in Exercise and Sport Science and Spanish, as well as a professional athlete competing with the USA women's national rugby team. In 2013, she earned a bronze medal at the Rugby 7s Women's World Cup in Moscow and competed in the 2014 15s World Cup in Paris and 2017 World Cup in Ireland. As an entrepreneur, former Harvard coach, and decorated professional rugby player, she loves sharing her knowledge through coaching and writing. Certified by the NSCA and Precision Nutrition, she brings her wealth of experience to the page, sharpening the lens by which we see the world. She writes for multiple small health and wellness businesses, as well as large publications such as Men's Health, MyFitnessPal, and EliteFTS. She now owns her own business, Dare Performance, in which she promotes a healthy lifestyle through journalism.

PHOTO CREDITS

Shutterstock.com: Pg. 1: Guas, 3: Rido, 6: Oleksandra Naumenko, 8: Jacek Chabraszewski, 10: Alexander Prokopenko, 12: Lucky Business, 14: CLS Digital Arts, 16: szefei, 18: photka, 20: Prostock-studio, 23: HQuality, 25: 3d_man, 27: GrAl, 28: Kateryna Kon, 30: bitt24, 32: siamionau pavel, 33: Elfhame, 35: SewCream, 37: Alena Ozerova, 39: Anna Hoychuk, 40: LifetimeStock, 42: Yulia Furman, 44: AlexLMX, 47: Dionisvera, 49: Joshua Resnick, 51: Zerbor, 53: Halfpoint, 55: Africa Studio, 56: Anton_dios, 59: ahalim, 60: Zerbor, 62: Alexander Prokopenko, 65: dimid_86, 66: Hannah Green Photography, 68: Inside Creative House, 70: Chad Zuber, 71: Maridav, 74: crystal light, 75: Daxiao Productions, 76: Syda Productions, 78: Monkey Business Images, 80: tolotola, 82: baibaz, 84: Vadim Martynenko, 86: PH888, 88: Luis Molinero, 90: Martin Novak.

EDUCATIONAL VIDEO LINKS

Chapter 1: http://x-qr.net/1Je4
Chapter 2: http://x-qr.net/1LQ4
Chapter 3: http://x-qr.net/1KrB
Chapter 4: http://x-qr.net/1KFe
Chapter 5: http://x-qr.net/1KJD
Chapter 6: http://x-qr.net/1KMr
Chapter 7: http://x-qr.net/1Lzh